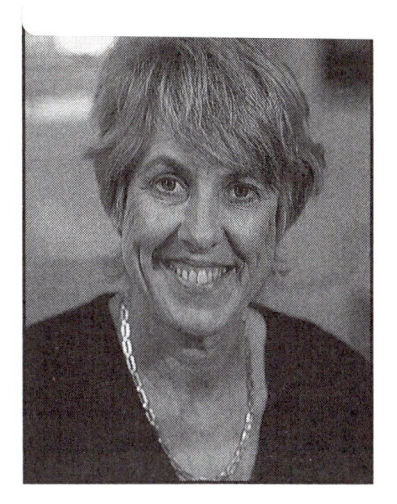

Scribe Publications
COMING OF AGE

Anne Deveson is a writer, broadcaster, and documentary film-maker. Her programs have won widespread recognition, including gold citations in the United Nations' Media Peace Prize, and awards for documentaries on social issues.

Her books include *Australians at Risk* (1978), *Faces of Change* (1984), and the best-selling *Tell Me I'm Here* (1991)—which won the 1991 Human Rights Award for non-fiction. In 1993, she was made an Officer of the Order of Australia for services to community health and to the media. She has been awarded honorary doctorates from the Universities of New South Wales and South Australia for services to the community.

Anne Deveson was born in June 1930, went to school in Australia, England, and Malaysia, was married for twenty years, and had three children. She now has a grown-up daughter and son, and lives near a ferry stop in Sydney with a fat dog, a thin cat, and too many telephone calls.

For Barbara Wace—mentor, friend, and intrepid traveller

*Anne Deveson*

# COMING
# of AGE

*Twenty-one interviews
about growing older*

SCRIBE PUBLICATIONS
NEWHAM AUSTRALIA

First published in Australia in 1994
by Scribe Publications Pty Ltd
RMB 3120, Lancefield Road
Newham Vic 3442

Copyright © Anne Deveson 1994

All rights reserved. Except as provided for by Australian copyright law, no part of this book may be reproduced without permission in writing from the publishers

Typeset in Galliard 10.5/13 by Scribe Publications
Printed in Australia by Australian Print Group

10 9 8 7 6 5 4 3 2 1

National Library of Australia
Cataloguing-in-Publication data:

Deveson, Anne, 1930– .
  Coming of age.

  ISBN 0 908011 28 8.

  1. Aged - Australia - Interviews. 2. Aged - Australia - Attitudes. I. Title.

305.260994

# Contents

| | | |
|---|---|---|
| *Acknowledgements* | | *vi* |
| *Introduction* | | *1* |
| 1 | **Mungo MacCallum** Divine discontent | 15 |
| 2 | **Ruby Langford Ginibi** Truth is what I'm about | 31 |
| 3 | **John Kingsmill** In place | 45 |
| 4 | **Freda Brown** My valuable wrinkles | 59 |
| 5 | **John Bray** I don't recommend it | 77 |
| 6 | **Colleen Clifford** I'm so lucky | 89 |
| 7 | **Bernard Lake** Making a choice | 99 |
| 8 | **Dorothy Buckland-Fuller** The wise ones | 113 |
| 9 | **Charles Birch** It's important to be excited | 127 |
| 10 | **Nell Forsdyke** I've had a lot of loving | 143 |
| 11 | **Leycester Meares** Never let anything go that you believe in | 153 |
| 12 | **Margaret Jones** Woman warrior | 163 |
| 13 | **Delys Sargeant** No wigs for our pubes | 183 |
| 14 | **Neville and Heather Bonner** At the top of the mountain | 197 |
| 15 | **Beryl Evans** I'm going to be a naughty old girl at ninety | 207 |
| 16 | **Bogdan Stojic** I'm 101. I will stop work. | 217 |
| 17 | **Carol Raye** Something our family is used to | 225 |
| 18 | **Tom Uren** Giving is the greatest form of loving | 237 |
| 19 | **Noreen Hewett** My life has been magnificent | 249 |
| 20 | **Dick Paget-Cooke** Bloody marvellous! | 259 |
| 21 | **Barbara Wace** I find the world terribly interesting | 268 |

# Acknowledgements

My thanks to Henry Rosenbloom of Scribe for suggesting this idea in the first place, and for his patience and thoughtfulness. Thanks also to the New South Wales Office on Ageing, particularly to Helen Leonard who is always a fund of information and support; and to Jenya Osborne and Hamish Campbell for their unflagging help and ideas. The quotation from Simone de Beauvoir on the opposite page is reproduced by kind permission of the publishers, Penguin Books.

I thank Sioned Fay and Jenniffer Atchison for their generous and creative contribution of most of the photographs. My thanks also to Penny Ramsay, who took the photograph of John Bray; Ponch Hawkes [Delys Sargeant]; Rochelle Franks [Bernard Lake]; Margaret Leggatt [Nell Forsdyke]; Shay Ryan [the Bonners]; and Edwin Webb [Barbara Wace].

Above all, I want to express my gratitude to the people I interviewed. They were generous with their time, courageous in their honesty, and thoughtful and humorous about their experiences of growing old.

*In old age we should wish still to have passions strong enough to prevent us turning in upon ourselves. One's life has value so long as one attributes value to the life of others, by means of love, friendship, indignation, compassion ...*
Simone de Beauvoir in **'Old Age'**


*When I grow up I wanna be an old woman.*
Michelle Shocked

# Introduction

I AM VERY OLD. I sit in a small room watching the rain beat down on sodden trees, while a cat yawls at my feet. The cat appeared unbidden on the day I arrived, and has lost much of its hair and most of its teeth. It smells. I am none of these things, and so I would like to kick the cat because I am here to finish this celebratory book about old age and not to be reminded of decrepitude. I grudgingly inject the cat with antibiotics. The first time, the needle passes through the animal's skin and out the other side into my thumb. I receive the antibiotics. It does not please me.

I read books about age and ageing, and listen to opera music which I play very loudly. The rain is relentless, and the grapes are falling in bruised purple heaps before they can be harvested. I sleep in a room with a Madonna that glows in the dark. In the kitchen are small plastic Madonnas full of water. I am not sure if this is holy water or ice-cubes.

In my reading, I am exploring the biology of ageing. My taste buds are declining, bone-loss accelerating, kidneys and bladder packing up, body fat piling on, discs shrinking, tendons stiffening. I am deeply depressed. I came to Italy because I felt it was timely to go away to write this book, to enter the portals of ageing, and to return somehow wiser and more resolved. Right now, I feel that the desert of my remaining days lies ahead, and I shall probably have to crawl across it. I will be a crabby old lady, and spiteful.

An owl falls down my chimney. It is an old owl, says the vet. A noble old owl. A beautiful noble old owl. We all stroke the tawny speckled feathers of the beautiful noble old owl, and I wonder why the owl is noble, the cat is not, and old people are often considered repugnant. Why can an ancient building crumble away and still be considered beautiful; but if we start crumbling away, nobody gathers round to say, 'Ah, che bella!'?

I am not yet into the obituary club: 'Have you seen old Fred is dead?' And I avoid those chilling roll-calls: 'John is weaker and needs more hoists, Fred has prostate cancer, Harriet has a polyp in her cervix, and Jane suffers from diabetes.' But depression is settling and, for me, this is unfamiliar.

I go for a walk on my brother's farm; he and his wife have lived in this region for many years. He is fifteen years younger than I; he is not very old. We squelch in brown mud through woods where there are mushrooms and truffles and golden salamander. At the top of a hill, I realise that, on the way up, I have been clinging onto tree trunks and branches. I fear that my balance is going. I might have osteoporosis. I might fall. I might break a hip. That would be the end. My brother is looking at me with incredulity. He is laughing. He gives me a big shove and I half fall, half race down to the bottom of the hill, and then collapse with laughter. I shout with joy. I am not old, I am young, young, young!

I race home and give the cat its injection. The cat sits on my lap for the first time. Its mange is improved, its breath is tolerable, it purrs.

Its name is Vittorio.

French author, Georges Simenon began feeling old when he was nearing sixty. He was depressed about whether he could ever escape Inspector Maigret and all the characters he had created in nearly two hundred novels. A few years later, after he had worked through his depression, he produced a book called *When I was Old*. 'Soon I shall be sixty-seven, and I have not felt old for a long time,' he wrote.

Simenon's experience, and mine, are examples of how easy it is to catapult ourselves into old age. Employers, in a depressed job market, can tell forty-year-olds they are too old—which means too old for them, thank you very much. If someone tells you that often enough, you will become old. Belief affects biology.

Children and adolescents often view us as old when we think we are still in the bloom of life. 'Are you very old? asked my four-year-old, when I was in my thirties. 'No,' I said. 'Good,' he replied. 'You still smell quite fresh to me.'

And how many of us have felt deeply old on landmark occasions, like first dates, and decade birthdays? I felt *very* old at the age of sixteen when, unbeknown to my parents, I met a friend in the Ritz Hotel for afternoon tea and solemnly puffed away at a cigarette through the veil of my mother's hat. The waiter was discreet; he did not suggest that I might set myself on fire.

So, what do we mean by old? Almost everybody in this book says they do not *feel* old, and there are countless anecdotes of people denying that it is their age that slows them up—it is their rheumatism or their arthritis. Strictly speaking, this is probably true. These are generally the people who say they haven't the time to be old, like 96-year-old Colleen Clifford (see page 89).

We are ageing from the moment of birth. When Dylan Thomas exalts in his poem *Fern Hill*, 'Now as I was young and easy under the apple boughs', he then jabs in a reminder that it isn't going to last for ever:

> Time held me green and dying
> Though I sang in my chains like the sea.

Numbers of people from post-modernists to new-age gurus are now challenging us to move outside the bounds of linear time in considering age. They ask, what do we mean by age? Chronological? Biological? Psychological? Chronological and biological do not always coincide. Ageing, says the American gerontologist Howell, 'is not a simple slope which everyone slides down at the same speed. It is a flight of irregular stairs down which some journey more quickly than others.'

Physician Deepak Chopra, author of several best-selling books on the mind-body relationship, presents the notion in *Ageless Body, Timeless Mind*, that old age, infirmity, and death are all 'in the mind' and are manifestations of the hypnosis of social conditioning. Buddhism also holds that life and death are in the mind. These are philosophical beliefs—Chopra and others would also say they are scientific—but it is hard to escape from corporeal identities when our knees ache or our hips give way.

We do not grow old in laboratories. We grow old in families or tribes, in cities or villages, alone or with others, in conditions of wealth or poverty, in environments that profoundly influence the way we age. And environments today are markedly different from our predecessors'.

Simone de Beauvoir, in her splendid and scholarly book, *Old Age,* shows how social and political factors strongly influence a society's attitude to age. In earlier societies, few people survived beyond their middle years—in ancient Greece, the average age of death for males was thirty—so that those who did grow old were likely to be highly revered and probably wealthy. Poverty and disease took an early toll of everyone else. Until the nineteenth century there was not even mention in historical records of the 'aged poor'.

De Beauvoir also shows that in those societies which were based on tradition and stability, such as ancient China in the Confucian era, the wisdom of old people was highly valued. But once a society became unstable, the most highly valued of its citizens were those who could fight their enemies and keep up with changing times. Age gave way to youth. For example, the decay of stable government in the Roman Empire soon led to the collapse of privilege for old people, and eulogies were replaced by satire—like this piece of savagery from the Roman satirist Juvenal:

> What a train of woes—and such woes—comes with a prolonged old age. To begin with, this deformed, hideous, unrecognisable face; this vile leather instead of skin; these pendulous cheeks; these wrinkles like those around the mouth of an old she-ape as she sits scratching in the shady Thabarcan woods ...

In century after century, going back long before the birth of Christ, unhappy old men bewailed their infirmities:

> How hard and painful are the last days of an aged man! He grows weaker every day; his eyes become dim, his ears deaf; his strength fades; his heart knows peace no longer; his mouth falls silent and he speaks no word ... all his bones hurt.
> —*Egyptian philosopher and poet, Ptah-hotep in 2500 BC*

Four-and-a-half thousand years later, Irish poet William Butler Yeats expressed similar views:

> What shall I do with this absurdity—
> O heart, O troubled heart—this caricature,
> Decrepit age that has been tied to me
> As to a dog's tail?

Yeats was so obsessed by the waning of his sexual powers that he had an operation to restore them, which led irreverent colleagues to call him, 'the gland old man.' But then the early Egyptians were also concerned to recapture youth: a papyrus reads, 'The beginning of the book on the way of changing an old man into a young one.' It advises the eating of fresh glands taken from young animals. In ancient Rome, elderly men were said to enter the Colosseum to drink the blood of dying gladiators because they believed it would ward off old age and death. Nowadays, most people wishing to snatch a few more years of youth opt for the surgeon's knife, collagen injections, plastic-foam implants, ray therapy, acids, or plain old abrasion. Plus ça change.

In historical writings, mention of women—particularly older women—is scarce. Women, both young and old, were invisible. Women lacked power, lacked education, and those that survived childbirth were frequently crippled by osteoporosis. At thirty, most women were considered old. Harsh living environments accelerated ageing and brought premature death for both women and men. But, because these were the only conditions that people knew, ravaged bodies were accepted as a part of life. Early photographs show stooped and emaciated bodies, receding jawlines where teeth had been pulled or fallen out, and sunken eyes. Depression killed the spirit before death killed the body. We have only to view current horrors in Africa to see how a child of twelve can become like an old man.

Today, we live in a new era in the history of ageing. In Western countries since the turn of this century, we have increased the average life-span of women and men in an unprecedented and astounding way. In 1900, the average life expectancy was forty-six years for women and forty-five years for men. Today, thanks to improved living conditions and medical progress, we live to a remarkable eighty years for women and seventy-four years for men. The average life expectancy for Aboriginal people is, shamefully, about twenty years less.

As a consequence of people living longer and having fewer children, the world's population is progressively ageing. By the year 2011, more than one in five of Australia's population will be aged sixty years and over. People over eighty years are expected at least to treble in numbers by the twenty-first century, and centurions such as Bogdan Stojic (see page 217) will no longer be a rarity. Australia remains locked into an ageing population—a trend that cannot be reversed, even if immigration remains high, and having more than two children comes back into vogue.

What does this mean in a society that has traditionally valued youth over age? Will the pendulum swing, as governments grow increasingly concerned about the financial, social, and political impact of ageing populations? Already, the Western world is spawning ministries and departments on ageing in a fevered bid to encourage independence till death do us part. Middle-aged people glumly prophesy that, by the time they are old, social security pensions for the aged will be but a dim and distant memory. Yet, at present, government pensions are the primary source of income for over three-quarters of people over the age of sixty-five. (Not that the old age pension allows for wine and roses: it generally amounts to about one-quarter of the average male wage.) Such attention from governments is welcomed, provsided older people are consulted. A rapidly growing industry is emerging of experts on ageing—health professionals, social workers, statisticians, architects, media strategists, public servants, social scientists, and therapists of varied hue.

Growing numbers of old people, better off and better educated than their parents and grandparents, offer a glory box of untapped markets to business, spurred on by 'grey market' research. Levi jeans now come in loose fit, and liposomes replace Ponds Night Cream, according to a joyously satirical article in the *Sydney Morning Herald* by Deirdre Macken. And June Allyson rides a golf buggy across our television screens, praising the efficacy and comfort of geriatric incontinence pads.

'New old age' proponents, such as Deepak Chopra and Betty Friedan, in her book, *The Fountain of Age*, develop passionate arguments that life after forty-five can be a new and wonderful experience for us all. We have the probability of one-third or even one-half more years of life than our ancestors—but, according to Friedan, only if we break through the 'age mystique' which hobbles us in age in much the same way she saw the feminine mystique hobbling women throughout life. Friedan uses a powerful metaphor when she maintains that, just as darkness is defined as the absence of light, age is currently defined as the absence of youth—downhill all the way to incontinence, senility, and the nursing home. She argues vehemently for 'acceptance, affirmation and celebration.'

If we are to redefine age, one of the prime areas of attention are mass media that are both sexist and ageist. In a patriarchal society where, historically, images of women are images that men like to look upon, older women fare particularly badly. They are either rendered invisible by having a 'use by' date, or they are required to compete in the youth stakes, with the patronising compliment, 'Isn't she marvellous!'

Television newscasters and models who survive past the age of forty rate breathless accolades in the women's press. Only the soaps offer scope for older women, perhaps because many of the most successful—such as *Golden Girls*—emanate from the United States where grey power carries clout.

Stereotypes and myths about old age which need debunking are those suggesting that old people are unproductive, physically decrepit, dependent on others in daily life, and incapable of learning. In fact, most older people today are healthy, productive, financially independent, and more likely to be giving care than receiving it. A recent study by the Institute of Family Studies found that three out of four older people provided child-minding help for their adult children, as well as emotional support in times of crisis; and four out of ten provided financial help.

Despite the common perception of people reaching their sixties, and then rapidly going downhill, the greatest physical decline occurs between the ages of thirty and forty years. Limiting chronic conditions increase only after seventy years. No differences in learning capacities appear until after seventy years, and then not appreciably until after ninety years. Observing the slogan 'use it or lose it' pays off. Chopra's *Ageless Body, Timeless Mind* tells of a gerontological study at Tufts University where the frailest residents were put on a weight-training regime: within eight weeks, wasted muscles had improved by 300 per cent, co-ordination and balance were better, and people who had not been able to walk unaided could now get up and go to the bathroom in the middle of the night by themselves. What made this accomplishment truly wondrous was that the youngest person was eighty-seven and the oldest ninety-six.

Then there's the hoary old chestnut that in Australia most old people are dumped into homes and forgotten. Nine out of ten people aged sixty years and over live in houses and flats, like the rest of the community, and most of them own their own homes. Even the majority of those old people who have significant handicaps live in the community with someone they know.

Tallying up the good news, the majority of people in Australia over sixty report that they are happy, and have satisfactory family and social lives. I suppose they could be more ebullient about it: they could say 'joyous'. But maybe such words are not part of a researcher's repertoire and, anyway, who is joyous all the time?

Being happy includes having good sex lives. Delys Sargeant (see page 183) deals with sexuality and ageing, a subject which in the minds of many young people is still viewed with incredulity. 'You don't!' they say. 'You aren't!'. Sex can flourish happily even into the nineties; but the subject of eroticism in old age has been aired so little that the old myths remain, including the one that desire disappears with age. What nonsense. Observe the flirtations between old people, read books like Gabriel Garcia Marquez' *Love in the Time of Cholera,* or Dorothy Hewett's *The Toucher,* about the passionate love between Esther La Farge, sixty-seven, and confined to a wheelchair, and Billy Crowe, young enough to be her grandson. Another lusty celebration of passion is found in Joyce Cary's *The Horse's Mouth*, in which ageing Gully Jimson, bad citizen, good artist, meets an old lover, Sara. He sees her first—ungallantly—as a 'fat old char with grey hair and a red face, breathing beer and suds.' But then, as she walks away, he finds a spark in the ashes: 'Amidst the lustful fire he walks; his feet become like brass. His knees and thighs like silver, and his breast and head like gold. Old Randipole Billy on the ramp. Embracing the truth.'

We are on a cusp, moving (as always) from one extreme of attitude and behaviour to another. Once, old people were savaged by rejection and neglect. Now, they are endangered by a relentless optimism which, while admirable, might well bring about feelings of real inadequacy. Not all of old age is super-smooth: there are some real downers, such as losing life-long friends and feeling, 'Is my turn coming next?' Or coping with illness which—yes, I know—isn't confined to old people, but comes with increasing incidence as parts wear out. So I have a sneaking sympathy with John Bray (see page 77) when he says about old age, 'I don't recommend it.' Or Earl Attlee, who grunted on his eightieth birthday that it was better than the alternative.

I don't know how I shall feel when I am eighty. But I am darned sure that it's as important to be as honest about our fears and feelings of inadequacy as it is to shout, 'Whoopdey-doo, I'm having a wunnerful time.' Friedan, who says that at the age of seventy-two she has 'never felt so free', was herself terrified and angry about old age when, twelve years earlier, she embarked upon writing *The Fountain of Age*. Sogyhal Rinpoche, Buddhist monk and author of *The Tibetan Book of Living and Dying,* surprised and relieved me when he admitted in an interview to his own fear of dying.

So let us be careful we don't swap one set of stereotypes for another which might be equally limiting. I, for one, don't want to be rolled in a marshmallow of euphemisms. I refuse to be known as a senior citizen, a tribal elder, or a golden oldie. I would loathe to end my twilight years in a sunset village. I do not want to be caring and sharing. And I am not growing older. I am growing old—a fact which I state quite mildly, but in protest against the saccharine brigade.

So that in Australia, where age is busting out all over, I make a plea (well, okay, a demand) for respecting differences. Some people will want to jump up and down on trampolines, or plunge into aquarobics. Others will choose to be isolates. Some will struggle with poverty or sickness that needs more than heated swimming pools to relieve the pain. Some will be mellow and benign; others will want to rant and rage. Some will join the soy-milk brigade; others might want to stuff themselves with chocolates and Stilton cheese. Didn't Noel Coward say, 'The secret of youth is a mixture of gin and vermouth'?

Common-sense also helps in dealing with ageing. Artist Margaret Olley says, 'Don't worry about face lifts. Let your mirror get dusty, then you can't see the wrinkles.' Others use humour. Scholar and writer John Bray departed from his more erudite poetry to produce these verses in *Quinquennial*:

> 'You must give up beer.'
> the doctor said
> 'Your weight is far too high
> You shouldn't want to go on drinking beer
> With sixty years gone by.
>
> 'Cigarettes are out,' the doctor said.
> 'If you want to stay alive.
> Your arteries are clogging up
> At the age of sixty-five.'
>
> 'Your prostate's got to go,
> The bloody thing's no good to you
> At seventy years or so.'
>
> Bereft of beer, of smokes, of sex,
> I only stay alive
> To see what else they'll rip off me
> When I turn seventy-five.

And French writer, Collette, in her last and most beautiful book, *The Blue Lantern*, chose to write an account of her final years when, although crippled with arthritis and largely confined to her room, she shows a wondrous capacity to find beauty and delight in the smallest of experiences: the shape and curve of her blue lantern; a seed pod which expels a delicate silvery follicle; the sound of children playing in the square. She even finds fascination in her pain—'pain ever young and active, instigator of astonishment, of anger ... the pain that enjoys an occasional respite but does not want my life to end: happily I have pain.'

Choice is important to self-respect, no matter how small or trivial the matter. In one of the interviews in this book—with Leycester Meares (see page 157)—I refer to the 'jelly' incident, which I witnessed while I was filming a documentary on disability several years ago. An eighty-year-old woman in a nursing home did not want custard with her jelly. She wanted 'just jelly.' The nursing attendant refused to oblige, snapping, 'Be a good girl and eat what you're given.' These infantilising and controlling behaviours are what people most dread as they grow old.

Sometimes we deny choice to old people, not because we are heartless but because we, not they, are the ones who cannot cope. A small old man, who looks like a ruffled and balding cockatoo, wants to stay in the room after his wife has just died. She had Alzheimer's. The nurse tries to move him out, in spite of his saying repeatedly, and like a gramophone record, 'But I want to stay, I want to stay.'

Somewhere along the way will come the moment that is inescapable: death. This is not a book about dying, except that the same principles of choice and dignity apply. My godmother, Yette, lived to ninety-four. She had suffered a series of strokes, and was lying apparently unconscious in her bedroom. The doctor stood in the doorway of the room and said to her daughter, in a matter-of-fact voice, 'You can let her die here, or have her taken to hospital.' From the frail little bundle in the bed there came a clear command. 'I choose to die at home,' she said firmly, and lapsed into unconsciousness again. She died at home.

Some of the people I interviewed for this book are friends; some, I did not know. I chose all of them because I thought their views would be interesting. I recorded the interviews at a time when I ruefully acknowledge that I needed to confront my own ageing. I remember standing in the London underground and seeing a poster, 'You can avoid the collecting tin, but you cannot avoid old age.' Instead of radiating joy or rushing to take out an insurance policy, I felt angry. I am not yet truly an 'integrated human bean,' as one child put it, and I am still trying to persuade myself that ahead of me lie golden ponds. Sometimes I can spy them; sometimes not. Occasionally, they are black bogs. But I am aware of the delights of liberation, the kind that led Jenny Joseph to write this much-read poem:

> When I am an old woman, I shall wear purple
> With a red hat which doesn't go, and doesn't suit me,
> And I shall spend my pension on brandy and summer gloves
> And satin sandals, and say we've no money for butter.

I observed a similar kind of freedom in my father, Douglas, who had lung cancer when he was seventy, and from then on changed his attitude to life. From inside a withdrawn and often disappointed man exploded someone of joyful eccentricity who climbed the Swiss alps, surfed at Bondi, lined his room with second-hand books three deep, and drove an old London taxi cab reciting poetry and singing Victorian music-hall ballads.

Truly, we undertake heroic journeys: often stumbling, sometimes flying, sometimes stagnating. Along the way, we experience emotions of passion, rage, indifference, jealousy, generosity—we encounter them all. If we allow ourselves, we will catch fire with the beauty of this world; a beauty that was expressed in blazing clarity by English writer Dennis Potter, three months after being told he only had a few weeks to live:

> The only thing you know for sure is the present tense; and that nowness becomes so vivid to me that, in a perverse sort of way, I'm almost serene. I can celebrate life. Beneath my window in Ross— Ross-on-Wye—when I am working the blossom is out in full. It's a plum tree ... it's the whitest, frothiest, blossomest blossom that there ever could be. And things are both more trivial than they ever were and more important than they ever were, and the difference doesn't seem to matter ... the glory of it, the comfort of it, the reassurance ... not that I'm interested in reassuring people—bugger that.

'Bugger that', he says, deflating his own saintliness. The man is translucent in his honesty, and that is how we best celebrate our lives. I don't think we are all cut out to be tribal elders—bugger that, too. Some old people are wise; some are foolish; some are interesting; some are downright bores. But, almost certainly, those who reach old age experience lives of extraordinary richness. In some, the richness is boldly seen. In others, it comes from small domestic happenings, stitched together year after year. There will be good stories and bad. Wolves eat grandmothers. Dragons can kill St George. St George can run away. But what a glorious sum of human experience. It shines from the stories people told me in this book. And that richness, that long journeying, is the beauty and the celebration of age.

*Anne Deveson*
Sydney, August 1994

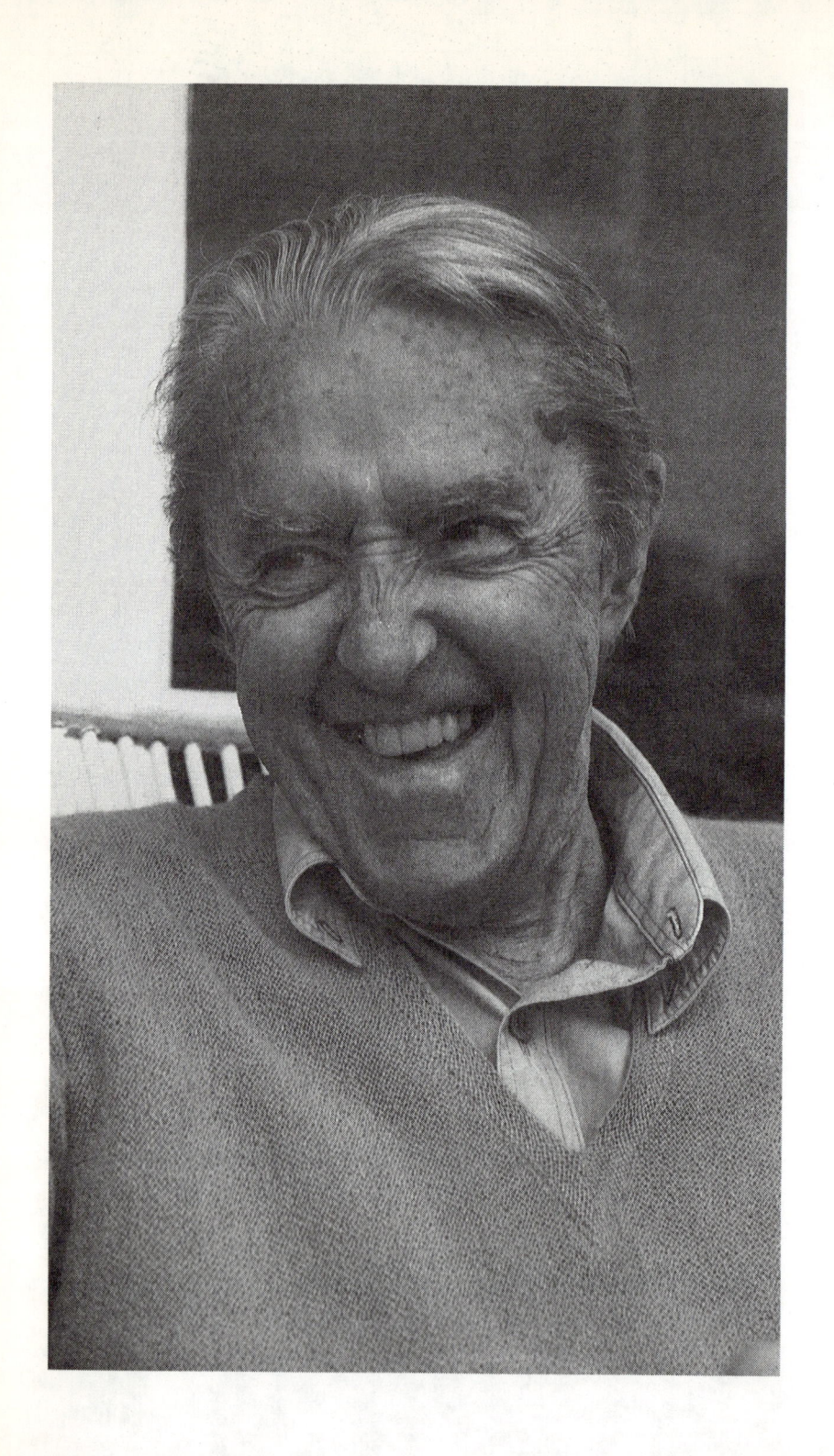

# Mungo MacCallum
*Divine discontent*

Mungo MacCallum, journalist, broadcaster, novelist and poet, disarms through gentle self-deprecation. He was born in Sydney in December 1913, educated at Sydney Grammar and the University of Sydney, worked for nine years on the staff of the *Sydney Morning Herald* and, during the war, was founder-editor of the Australian Army Journal *Salt*. After the war, he was a columnist on the Sydney *Sun*, undertook lecture tours with Britain's department of information in the United Kingdom and the Mediterranean, and became ABC features editor in 1950. He produced the historic opening night of ABC television in 1956, and made a distinguished contribution to radio and television broadcasting, specialising in the arts.

Later, he continued as a freelance writer and producer in both radio and television, and was television critic for *Nation*. He was runner-up in the British Commonwealth Jubilee prize for radio plays, and in the International Radio Prix Italia. He won the Australian Writers' Guild award in 1972 for the best script in any medium. He has published two novels, *A Voyage in Love* and *Son of Mars*, poetry in various journals and anthologies, and an autobiography, *Plankton's Luck*.

He has one son, Mungo IV, well known as a political writer and satirist. Mungo MacCallum lives in a Balmain house overlooking Sydney Harbour with his wife, Polly, who is a sculptor. Several times in the interview, he apologised for his wheeziness, saying somewhat crossly that it was because he had given up smoking—which made him feel much older.

Yes, it's true. It did make me feel older. It's now ten months, and I want it just as much. I went to this absurd hypnotherapist, and it was so banal it maddened me. He said all the nice things about how I'm giving up an old friend now after sixty years, and I must let that friend go, and then he made me lie down and talked the obvious clichés, and the two hours cost me $180. The second hour he'd had some very high cheese for lunch, and he breathed it over me. Here was I trying to be a good patient, and I was torn between laughter and fury. And it didn't make the slightest difference.

*Well, then, what did? Something worked.*
No, I still long for it every moment of every day.

*You'd think that, because you feel better, you'd therefore feel younger.*
I think it's because when you make such a radical change after sixty years—I'm in my eightieth year—it tends to tip you over into old age, just like having some sort of bereavement or an accident. It's obviously the thing to do, and I do feel that I'd be a fool if I started again. It has saved some money, I suppose, although I do want to drink more wine.

*Are you very often conscious of age?*
Yes, I am. I find the number eighty recurring in my mind all the time. Very strange. I try to keep on working, and I have done quite well. It's not something I'm frightened of, but it's something that is there. Just like waking up in the morning and taking my sleeping pill at night before I go to sleep, it's there all the time.

*What does it mean to you when it's there?*
It means that I find it harder to do my exercises. I find myself stiffer— these are all the aches and pains of age, you know—and I have to try to stop myself going to the doctor every time when my back hurts, because I feel one mustn't become a hypochondriac. I try, in other words, to be more or less as normal. But I feel I've changed a lot, emotionally and physically and psychologically. I'm more fatalistic. I'm also much more silent. I don't talk nearly as much, believe it or not. I find I'm quite happy to sit at meals, and my wife Polly accepts this. If I have nothing to say, I don't say anything.

*This is something that I've observed in others. Is it because you're conserving energy?*

I think it's partly conserving energy because one does feel tired. I don't feel bouncy. It's also partly this business of 'been there, done that'. You know? We went the other night to see a French film, which was pretty well done; but I kept on saying to myself by about the middle, 'Far too long'. The way it was done, it was obviously going to be far too long. I don't want to be one of these people who think that nothing new is any good, because I think a lot of new things are marvellous—and that includes a lot of rock music. By the same token, it's so difficult when somebody's enthusing about something which you first experienced round about 1930, and you have to try to be part of that enthusiasm. When you're by yourself you don't have to be part of that.

*Are there things that do enthuse you?*

Oh, yes: fine performances of music, fine performances in the theatre, like that wonderful experimental English company that came out in the last Sydney Biennale, they did *The Street of Crocodiles*. By the same token, Polly and I were disappointed when we went to see *Dancing at Lughnasa*—that Irish thing which we thought was going to be pretty good; but it wasn't radical, it was just a well-made Irish play, no more than that. Apart from the theatre and music, I get tremendous thrills out of good film; good books, of course, both fiction and non-fiction; good poetry; interesting painting and sculpture; plenty of things like that. And nature can suddenly be wrenchingly beautiful or fascinating.

*In the notes you sent me, you said that you were not afraid of death or of dying, but you were afraid of losing your capacity for beauty.*

Yes. I know it sounds a bit pompous, but it is true, and I do find a lot of what people enthuse about now not beautiful. One can share these enthusiasms without being part of them. That's why I get on fairly well with young or youngish people, because I don't retreat into a crusty silence.

*Have you become more mellow or has the reverse happened?*

I'm not sure. As I said, I'm much more fatalistic—for instance about Australia—the 'great thing', the talking point about what we are, where we are going, I am fatalistic about that, but at the same time I'm frequently absolutely exasperated. It's a sort of divine discontent, mixed with spasms of content.

*Do people treat you differently?*
People who don't know me do. People occasionally get up and give me their seat in the bus, which I'm very glad of. It angers me, but I'm glad of it. And a lot of people call me 'Sir', which is surprising these days. By the same token, of course, a lot of people, meeting them for the very first time, like carpenters or plumbers or tradesmen, just call me Mungo—which is the opposite, the Australian way.

*Has your sense of family changed at all?*
I went on a bit about my family in my autobiography, but I said in the book that I reserve the right to change my mind; and I do think I've been a bit hard on them. But there were good reasons I thought at the time for keeping well away from my family, partly because of my terrible matriarchal German grandmother. But since then there's nobody except my son, and he lives well away from Sydney, right up near Queensland. I have two grand-daughters of whom I'm very fond, and who seem to be fond of me; and the one who is at university in Sydney is the one who rings up and says, 'Can I come and see you?' I feel it's nice, but I don't feel it's a great family thing. It's *wonderful* to have grand-daughters. When young Mungo was born I didn't feel this glow of achievement that so many fathers seem to feel, which I suspect is really a sort of self-pride.

*One of the characteristics I've always enjoyed about you is your sense of absurdity. Has that increased as you've got older?*
I don't think it's increased, but it's alive and well. I still find an extraordinary number of things absurd. Most of it's fantasy, and therefore I sometimes suspect that there is something slightly wrong with me; because if one sees so many things as absurd, and other people don't, is one a bit off kilter? Also, a sense of absurdity can be double-edged, become destructive cynicism. Or lead to stereotyping.

*Has it always been like that?*
Yes, always. It was part of my boyish dreams, how absurd things were. When I was at Sydney Grammar we used to go to these football matches on Saturdays. I was never any good at football, thank goodness, but the parents frequently used to come. I used to watch them, especially the men, walking around and talking to each other, little bubbles of cliché seemed to be coming out of their head, 'Well played, lad'. That

still happens. I still have these fantasies which are based on the truth, but they make the truth absurd.

*That must have made it difficult sometimes, working at the ABC!*
It certainly did. But, by the same token, there was such a burden, especially as one got sucked into the administrative stuff, that one didn't have much chance to laugh. One wanted more to rage. The early part was great—when I was with radio features, before television began—because then I was simply a programme writer and producer and editor. That was marvellous and after, when I was in charge of TV training and getting TV on the air; but the later administrative part was hell.

*Was most of your working life spent at the ABC?*
No. Before the war, I had to cut my residence at the University, at St Andrews College where all the family always went, because my father died and I got this cadetship on the *Sydney Morning Herald*. I'd not known what I wanted to be. I'd toyed with the idea of architecture, music, painting, all these things; and then suddenly I found myself on the *Herald*, and I found I enjoyed journalism. I enjoyed moulding things. Then the war came, and I tried to enlist in various ways and was always rejected with contempt. Finally, I was invited into the Army to start and run the Army journal *Salt*, and that was a success. At the end of the war, I came out with some sort of reputation which was ironic. I did a little more journalism and hated it; I went to England and did a lecture tour; came back; and was invited to join the ABC.

*Looking back, do you have a sense of having lived many lives?*
Variations on one life, more than many different lives. I know this sounds a bit pompous, but it's always had a creative root, in various forms. And for that reason sometimes one looks back and thinks, 'Well, I regret not having concentrated more on *one* form of creation, like painting, which Grace Cossington Smith wanted me to do; or music, which Mysie Stephen wanted me to do.' Perhaps it would have been better, but I don't really regret it. It's been a variegated sort of a life. It's lasted quite a long time, and one's had one's moments of extreme satisfaction.

*Has age affected your creativity?*
I think recently, since I stopped smoking, it's slowed me down. I find

things come more slowly, and I forget things. I might have an idea and I'll give it a key word, a mnemonic so that I won't forget it, and then when I come around to think what it was, I've forgotten the key word. I think the imagination's in fairly good form, partly because of this absurdity faculty—even though it doesn't always come out in the writing. But otherwise I do think I'm—well, I am slower.

*Does this irritate or depress you?*

Yes. Very much. The trouble is, you see, the time that one saves by not automatically reaching for cigarettes doesn't happen—I still automatically do this when I'm trying to think of something—so I lose the time and I don't get the thought. It's all part of just getting bloody old, that's it.

*What about your physical appearance? As a young man were you vain; were you narcissistic?*

I was narcissistic, but not vain. I just cannot bear to shave. I had to force myself this morning, because I'm so sick of seeing my face in the mirror. I didn't realise for years until a friend who was much older said, 'You are *fascinated* by your own emotions.' Which is absolutely true. It's not a *vain* fascination. It's just that, without realising it, I think, 'Gosh I'm very upset about this. Or I'm very ...' It's a sort of me-me-me thing. It's not a preoccupation; it just happens all the time without one's knowing.

*But what about not wanting to look at yourself in the mirror; what's going on there?*

I think it's because I've been doing it for eighty years. I'm sick to death of doing it. And also I find my look, my eyes, irritate me in some sort of way. Once somebody said to me, 'You have very frightening eyes.' And I said, 'Why?', and she said, 'They look through me.' I think it was because I was thinking about the emotion that she produced in me. But it's just that I'm tired of seeing myself.

*Do you get any pleasure out of being able to get away with things now that you couldn't when you were younger?*

There've been so many times in my life when I've behaved terribly badly, because I've been drunk, that the outrageousness is passé—as far as I'm concerned. Now I very seldom am outrageous. I don't get any pleasure out of it. I always feel sorry afterwards if I have been. Recently, we went to lunch with somebody who had a much-touted house in the country, and I hated the place. It was claustrophobic; it was right at the bottom of a very steep dark valley; we didn't have lunch until about four o'clock in the afternoon; and I wasn't drinking anything. Later, they came here, and Polly said afterwards that I'd been far too frank. I didn't think I had. They hadn't taken offence, but I don't feel I want to get away with anything any more. I am perhaps a bit less wild than I used to be, because it was a wild sort of angry drunkenness, and now it's not. I care less and I try to be polite.

*You have written and talked about the joy that you have from your marriage with Polly. Has getting older affected that?*
Well, one is ... less demonstrative. She undoubtedly saved my life, even though neither of us thought of it as that, at the time. I was in the depths of depression, and I'd had a pretty rough ten years. She was like a lifeline to me, and I think the marriage has stayed that way. There's not so much passion in it, and I think it's rather like most marriages as they get by. It's affection and companionship.

*That comes across strongly—that, and a shared humour. Looking back into your childhood, were you conscious of old people around you?*
I became highly conscious of this matriarchal grandmother quite soon, because we lived cheek by jowl. There was this ghastly set-up where the grandparents had very generously built a house for my newly married mother and father in their garden, and it came to seem to me a fatal thing to do. Grandfather was a very nice jolly fellow, very kind and very generous, and very full of jokes. We used to have these reading sessions on winter Sunday afternoons. I remember the Scottish burr; and the purr of the gas fire in the grate; and reading Sir Walter Scott, who was the most enormous bore. But it all seemed to fit in perfectly, and grandfather was always very good as far as I was concerned.

*And grandmother?*
Grandmother took everything over. She ran the family. I didn't like her, and I liked her even less when, shortly after I got married to Diana Wentworth and I was twenty-six and on the *Sydney Morning Herald* doing very well, I took Diana to meet her just as a courtesy. With a

sweet smile, she said, 'What a pity you've ruined his career by marrying early. He was doing so well.' That didn't endear me to her, and also the fact that I thought she treated father badly, which may have been part of his tragedy. I was told that, from the age of twelve, father had never cost his parents a penny. Scholarships and a brilliant student and Rhodes scholar, the lot. Never once had she given him an encouraging word, and I thought, 'Well, fuck you.'

*Your mother lived until she was 101. Were you close?*
I found her mysterious and ... this is another injustice that I did. Because of the experience with grandparents and how they'd been too close to my parents, I was determined when I married Diana that I wouldn't subject my wife to that set-up. In fact, an uncle of mine said to my wife before we were married, 'Don't forget, you'll be marrying the family.' It made me the more determined, and that meant that I paid far too little attention to my mother; and she was a wonderful mother, just as my father was a wonderful father. She never complained. They always gave everything that they could. There was no whimsy. There was no chance of our expanding ourselves that was ignored; they did everything for us without spoiling us.

At the same time, mother was a product of the nineteenth century. She was very much of the order that men were superior: one didn't query them; one didn't talk about them; and so on. I didn't ever really get to know her. Yet she had a lot of young friends, they adored her, and they knew her far better than I did. When she died, one of these friends, by then a middle-aged woman, said to me she was the most wonderful mimic—which I'd never known. And also that she was 'the most stoical woman that I have ever met'. This is what this woman said—and I suddenly realised, by God she was. She'd had all the family die except me, all in tragic circumstances, and she'd never complained. She'd never said how lonely she was, she was a mystery to me, and that's one thing I do feel guilty about.

*Did this affect your attitudes later to women, do you think? Did you have this sense of distance from other women?*
Maybe so. I'm not sure. I know this sounds incredibly naive and romantic, but I've always thought there was a sort of mystery about women, and it wasn't simply the physiological and biological mysteries. I was afraid of being the intrusive, insensitive male. It seemed to me

that they were different 'beings' from men. I think it's a difference of nature not of nurture. I know that does sound absurd and romantic—I think it may have been an offshoot of my attitude to mother.

*What did your mother look like? What were your memories of her at the time you were growing up?*
There's a little photo there—this was when she was married.

*Oh, she was beautiful.*
Yes.

*Was she affectionate?*
Yes, she was extremely affectionate. But here again I think I flinched away from it a bit. Also, by the same token, I don't think she or my father talked to each other enough. When I see families nowadays saying, 'Go and get stuffed, Mum,' I think we were very tight-lipped. The first occasion I remember that I got really pissed, when I was about eighteen, and I was carried home and woke up next morning on the sofa in the study, she didn't say anything. Oh yes she did. She said, 'You were very tired last night.' It's just extraordinary, I think. I have no idea what she thought about the vast bulk of things.

*And with your father?*
It was the same, although in his case he had this frightful accident; and he became a huge drinker, a very quiet but huge drinker. He was offered this wonderful, glittering prize at Oxford just as a graduate, which was very unusual. He was offered the Chair of Law, and refused it; and came back, set up as a barrister, and wasn't allowed to go to the war. He was told that he had to stay and read letters, decode ciphers and things. As a result, after that war there was a huge pro-veteran thing, and he didn't get his practice going, with the result that he became terribly ... terribly sad. And then he had this awful accident, his hand, which was agonising for years.

*What actually happened for those years?*
He loved bicycling in the country, and he used to go off for the weekend. One weekend he came back on Sunday night and gashed his hand, he said, and thought nothing more of it. By Monday, he was fighting for his life. In those days there were no antibiotics, and he had operation

after operation. The hand was cut open over and over and over again, and by the time they'd finished he was too weak even to have an anaesthetic, and the hand was like that for the rest of his life. He had to write with his left hand, and he was in constant pain. I think, what with one thing and another, the disappointment of his unlikeable mother and the law thing at Oxford—although he chose to come back—and all the rest of it ... There is a predisposition in our family to be drunk, there's no doubt about that. He was; I was; my sister was; and ... I mean, I know it's not an excuse, but I think it's partly a biological thing as well as partly a temperamental thing ...

*At what stage do you think that you first became conscious of getting older? Can you remember a moment or a time?*
Eighteen [laughter], when I first had my huge drunk, and I realised this was going to happen for the rest of my life. In the other sense, I honestly don't know. People say that with men, when they become forty, they suddenly realise they've reached a turning point. I didn't. 'Over the hill' was the phrase that use to be used, at forty. Even at sixty, seventy, I've been conscious of this; but not until now has my age of eighty clanged in my ears.

*When your mother was in her nineties, and indeed when she was 100 or 101, what was she like then?*
She was pretty good until the last few years. She was always courteous, very sweet, and her nurses all loved her. She was very very frail, and gradually lost sight, lost hearing, lost just about everything. And then in the last very few years, we had to put her in a nursing home; it was too difficult. She herself, even before then, was saying, 'Dears, do let me go into a nursing home.' And finally we did. She became wafty, and then just a tiny little ... shrivelled, bent ... thing.

*Would you like to live as long as she did?*
Not under those conditions. But there was that woman in the paper the other day who was a hundred, and pretty jolly with it, you know.

*You might be able to take up smoking again when you're a hundred.*
Yes. Yes, maybe I'll do that on my eightieth birthday. No, unless one was in reasonably hale and intelligent health, I don't think so—not live as long as she did.

*What about if you were able now to get an extension of life as you are now—given the remarks you made about ennui, would you like to go on in perpetuity?*
I think so, because so far, the sense of discovery or interest outweighs the ennui. But for how long I should go on, heaven knows. I can't imagine, say, living twenty more years, and sustaining the same amount of enthusiasm as I have now. I don't think it's physically possible for a lot of people. For a few people it is, like that old woman the other day. After a certain point, I think that to live on unchanged involves an innate simplicity, a limited horizon. It's very hard to imagine, continuing totally unchanged, and that's one of the good things I think about life in the average way. You grow older imperceptibly. You don't suddenly wake up in the morning and find you can't move, or think, or speak, or something—unless you've had a stroke.

*Are you indeed not frightened of dying?*
Oh, I don't think I'm frightened. But I am frightened of a protracted, painful, or senile death. And I don't want to be a nuisance.

*Do you have any curiosity about what might happen after death, if anything?*
I'm convinced that nothing happens. It's not a problem, as far as I'm concerned.

*Have you always thought like that?*
In a more or less inchoate way, yes. But I'm convinced of it now. I'm convinced of the idea of 'A God', but not outside us. It's in us and ... everything one reads now—the Upanishads and all these things—they've all got this idea basically. It's only very naive people think that there's something, some*body* out there.

*So do you have any sense of some order or design of God within?*
I think there is an external sense of order, which I regard as a scientific thing, a primal, a primal cause; but not God. I think God is within in the sense that we conceive Him or Her or It as the hopeless model, for us in our better moments. And when we say, 'It's God's will,' we just mean *we* have failed or our friends or our enemies have won.

*Were you hard on yourself, in life, do you think?*
Polly says I am, still. I don't think so. I think I've been pretty self-

indulgent, actually. I know there is allegedly this Scottish strain, which may have linked up with my grandmother's Prussian strain to make a sort of grim accuser. I think I did have high standards, not of conduct but of performance—writing or broadcasting or whatever—but I don't think I'm hard on myself. Though perhaps I've paid a high price in guilt toward others.

*And in your writing now, are there areas that you still want to explore?*
Yes there are, but I'm not sure whether I'll get anywhere. I've just finished another novel. I published the autobiography in 1986, and it was short-listed for the *Age* Book of the Year. Before that, I'd been so busy with television and radio and so on, that I'd not published any novels for about twenty years, This one probably wouldn't be best-seller stuff, because they never have been.

*You might start a whole new cult.*
Yes. The worst seller [laughter].

*Mungo, how would you like to be remembered?*
Ah, this is very difficult. One either sounds narcissistic or arrogant. I'd like people to remember me with ... some affection, and I suppose, to an extent, with a little bit of admiration. I suppose so, yes. But that sounds arrogant. I think the point about it, really, is to remember that one is remembered fondly by those who are close to one; but, as the years go by, the works and the person gradually recede.

*Has getting older been a humbling experience or a liberating experience, or both?*
Both. One feels ... one can be accepted for what one is more, because now they'll say, 'Well, the old bugger can't change.' At the same time, it's been humbling insofar as you can't do things which you took for granted.

*I think I was picking up more there on that sense of the recognition that one's place in the world is very fleeting.*
Very fleeting, and the more so I meant when you take the really long view, which is that entropy will cause the universe to fall in on itself and there won't be the slightest memory of anything or anybody. But even in the short term, Shakespeare has been up and down in terms of

people's admiration several times. There are so many fashions in memory, it seems to me, quite apart from the quality of what's remembered. I think one would like to be remembered, but knows that it must be a fairly fleeting affair.

*Do you have any sense of meaning or purpose to your life?*
Not when one considers the inevitability of loss and decay, and so on. I think you have to put it in a little pod and say, within that pod, one tries to grow and to operate, and to be fruitful. But not long-term meaning. I think it's very easy to be cynical about humankind, but I also think it's reasonable to be cynical. I think we're pretty atrocious.

*Cynical in what way and for what reason?*
The hopelessness of humankind and its incorrigibility ... well, you've only got to look at the world now.

*But do you have any sense of any improvements?*
I think yes, but we cancel that out by being worse in other ways. I mean, someone said the other day about young people now: 'The good are better than they used to be; the bad are worse.' I think this is true about humankind generally. We advance with one step, and discover things and so on, and we abolish slavery; but with the other step we go back—we make people into slaves, and kill them and rape them.

*We pretend we don't now, though.*
It's only a pretence. There are lots of people of good will in the world, perhaps more than there used to be; but equally there are more people in the world who are suffering and have bad lives. I would say the Bush slogan was the latest of the big, new happiness slogans, and within minutes the whole of Yugoslavia is in flames, Cambodia, Somalia. I think there are fifty-two wars going on at the moment. And so how can you really say that more goodies are in a better situation than the baddies? I don't think they are.

*Does this affect you?*
Someone once wrote about 'the brilliance of despair'. I don't feel as bad as that. More a sort of fatalistic sorrow for mankind. It's easy to see why ancient peoples invented wilful gods to explain their own faults to themselves. It's very easy to retreat into a dead-end feeling and say,

'Oh well.' But I think one has to remember the whole time, yet try to keep on with one's own little work. By work, I don't mean charity or anything like that—but one certainly should help—but just to keep on as if life were good.

*And is it?*

I think on the whole it has been for me. You see, I've been so lucky. I've had the most fantastic life. Things have happened to me that should really have made me drop off ages ago—car smashes, and all sorts of terrible things—and I've been enormously lucky, both in that, and in personal relationships on the whole. And in being able to do the work I want to do. When you think of the enormous number of people who can't do the work they want to do, and who've got to scribble and scrabble the whole time to get by, I've been very lucky.

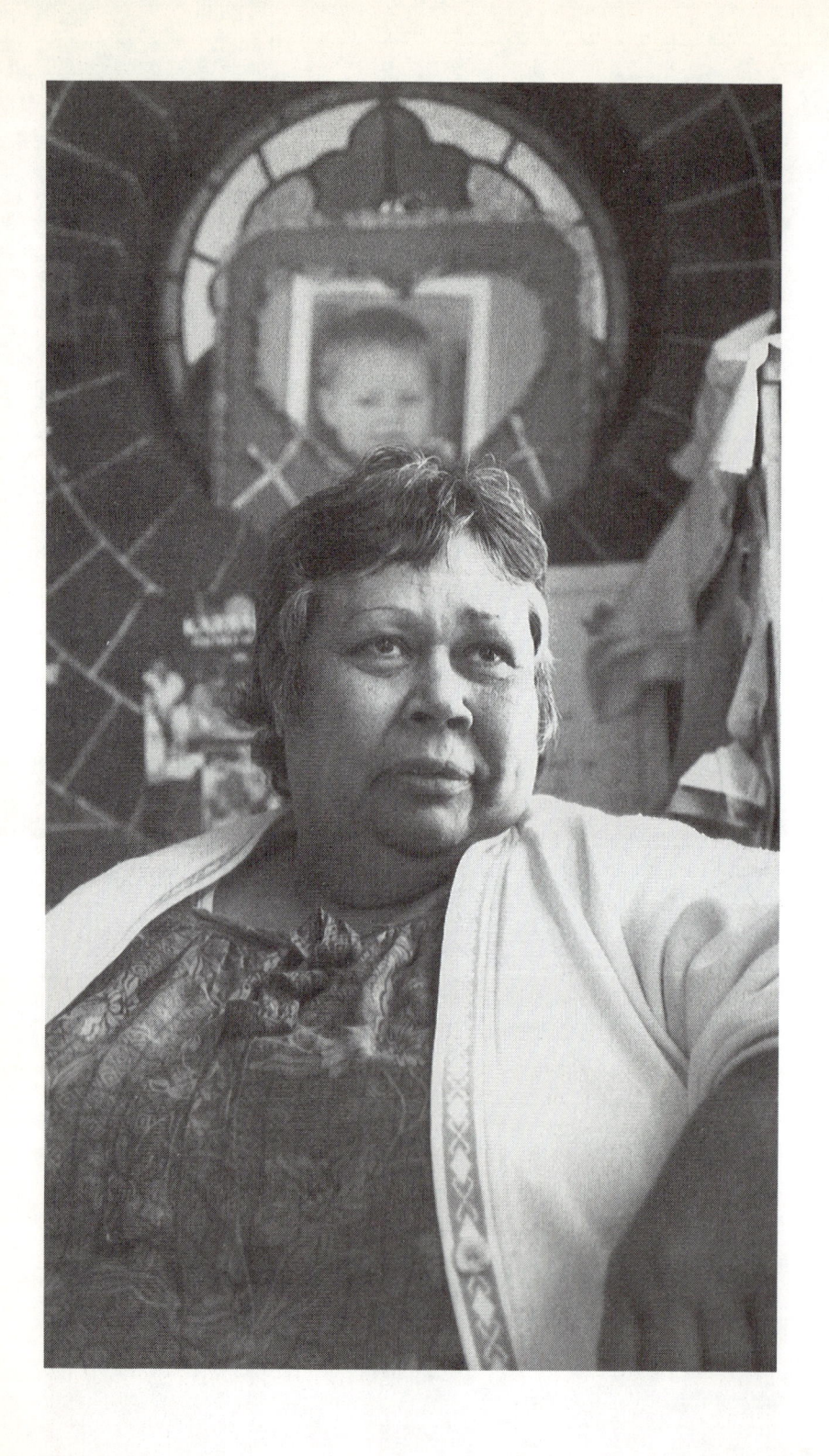

# Ruby Langford Ginibi
*Truth is what I'm about*

Ruby Langford Ginibi is a writer, and now spends much of her life researching the history of her people, the Bundjalung tribes. 'Writing is a way to the truth' she says. She lives in an Aboriginal hostel in Sydney, called *Allalwah*, which means 'Stop! Sit down and rest awhile.' Her large room is also her office, full of photographs, letters, newspaper cuttings, official records, paintings. She has diabetes, cancer, and arthritis, uses a walking frame, but still gets around—lecturing, researching, visiting her family.

Ruby was born in January 1934 at the Box Ridge Mission, Coraki, on the far north coast of New South Wales. She calls the date of her birthday, 26 January, 'shame day.' She was raised in Bonalbo, went to high school in Casino and, at age fifteen, moved to Sydney and worked as a clothing machinist. She has raised nine children—mostly by herself—and has twenty-one grandchildren. For many years, she lived in tin huts and camped in the bush around Coonabarabran, working at fencing, pegging roo skins, burning off, lopping, and ring-barking. Other times, she lived in the Koori areas of Sydney and worked in clothing factories.

She has written three books: her most recent, *My Bundjalung People*, was published in 1994; *Real Deadly* is a collection of short stories and poems; and her autobiography, *Don't Take Your Love to Town*, won a 1988 Human Rights Literature Award. Her fourth book, *Haunted Past—Nobby's Story*, will be about her eldest son, Nobby, who has spent almost half his life in gaol.

There's always been a difference in the way Aboriginal societies treat old people. In your Anglo societies, you have a triangle like this: the top controls the bottom, whereas in our societies you've got the bottom controlling the top. We had a very democratic system before the place was colonised. There were no kings and queens. We had tribal elders, the law-givers and, in traditional society, if you broke the law you were banished. I don't mean just for a couple of days—you were banished for ever. Otherwise, you were stood about in the flat, and then they threw a spear at you and, bang, you were gone. That was justice. But the old people and the young ones were the most loved and looked after. They always got the choicest cuts of the meat that the hunter brought. Our societies were based on sharing and caring; nobody was without. I think we were the first communists [chuckles].

*If you were an old person, did you automatically become an elder?*

Yes, because being an elder meant that you had more knowledge than the young people.

*And what about in urban life now, are old people still respected in Aboriginal societies?*

Of course. The old people are always respected, even in urban societies. This place that I live in is the first-ever hostel for older people. We've got a 103-year-old lady here, and our people don't usually live to that age. She used to muster cattle.

*You are an elder of your own tribe. What does that mean?*

I am an elder of the Bundjalung tribe, and I have been given my tribal name Ginibi by my tribal aunt. It means black swan. Big one!

*So do you keep in touch with your people?*

Yes. We've had a submission for some land to get a cultural centre for the young kids, because there's nothing there. These people have been dispossessed of everything. They live in two different societies up there. White fellows and Koories, they still don't come together. But the Koories still go hunting for bush tucker, and they fish, stuff like that. Bundjalung National Park is the place of a great massacre of my people from Box Ridge Mission, back in the 1840s. It's very sacred ground to our people. The old ones used to say to me, 'You can spend the day there, and have a barbecue, but don't go to sleep there because the old ones will torment you. They'll walk around you with their spears at night time and you won't sleep.' This is true. Even me, I would not go there unless one of our old ones came with me. It's a very sacred place; a lot of our people are from there. It should have been handed back to our mob a long time ago. And that's the way it is there.

*When you were growing up, do you remember some of the old people around you?*

Oh yeah, yeah, I remember the old ones there on the mission. Emma's sister, granny Mary, she used to look after me when I was a little girl. I was six, and Gwen my other sister was four, and Rita was two when our mother run off and left us. And I can remember in my mind's eye this old woman that looked after me. I went back after forty-eight years' absence, and I said to aunty Eileen, my father's sister, 'Can we go and talk to the old ones? She said, 'Oh, we don't bother the old ones. But if they're sittin' on the verandah, pull up when you go past.'

I was so anxious, because I thought I could remember this old woman—we were driving past, and I could see one old woman sitting on the verandah. So I said to my adopted girl, Pammy, 'Pull up, pull up.' And I ran to the fence, and I called out, 'Aunty, do you know me?'

She looked at me with these most piercing dark eyes you've ever seen—she's a full blood, you know.

'Who are you, girl?' she said.

'Ruby Anderson,' I called out.

And she sang out in lingo to another old one inside. Next minute, this head poked around the corner of the door: 'Who your father?'

And I said, 'Henry Anderson.'

She said, 'Your mother Evelyn?'

And I said, 'Yes.'

'You Ruby!'

I said, 'Yes.'

'Oh, my girl, come inside, don't you stand out there. I used to look after you when you was a little bebby. And I used to wash you and bath you. And next minute I look you'd be in the mud making mud-pie. I used to dress you up and make you pretty and keep you clean, and you used to cry all the time, and hang on to my dress. I couldn't get away from you.'

I just burst out crying. I ran in and sat on the verandah, and she brought a chair out and sat there. Next thing, there's aunty Eileen coming up the road with her little walking cane, and they all wore these beanie caps. There's the three elders up there and there's me. I just sat and held her hand, and I could feel the love coming through from that old girl. She died in February 1991, this old girl that used to look after me. She was 102. But oh, it was a loving experience.

I can remember the manageress of this mission where I was born, she ended up being the manageress of that infamous Cootamundra Girls Home. Her name was Mrs Hiscocks. Yeah, memories of that place were terrible—all written up in my book, *Don't Take your Love to Town*. How they used to hold our nose every Monday morning, and down would go a tablespoon of treacle or syrup and raw sulphur—it was a form of antibiotic. Bathing was in caustic soda and water, because you only had tank water and it was very precious, so all the water that was used for washing had handfuls of caustic soda chucked in it for the unbleached calico sheets and stuff. My memories of that place were no good.

Word would go round that the protection people were coming to take the kids. They started off by rounding up just the half-caste kids, mainly to hide the fact that they were fathered by white men. That is how we got our degrees of caste to begin with, you know. And then we'd hear. 'The Welfare's coming, the Protection's coming for the jarjums' (kids). You'd see them running and they'd hide 'em in the scrub, till they came and went, you see. All this stuff was going on. This is the sad history that this country knows nothing about. Some want to know and some don't.

But you can't do what has been done to a race of people like ours without having disastrous results. We have been divided, quartered, split apart and torn asunder by the powers that be, namely the governments of the day in this country. We've always had to conform to the standards of the invading people in this country; we've never been allowed to be our damned selves. We're still not allowed. We still don't have no power. We still don't have a voice either. Other people are writing our stories and giving their perspectives of us—anthropologists, academics, big-shot book writers who rip us off for the sake of the glorious buck—and how they write and perceive Aboriginal people perpetuates and keeps alive the racism and the stereotyping of my people in this country. It has to stop. Until we can have a say about what affects us in this country, we don't have no human rights. There's a lot to be heard.

*Is this what keeps you going—because you've been very ill?*
Oh love, I'm not dead yet. Don't write me off. There's a very strong Koori spirit behind this old woman. Yes, I have never been so motivated in my damned life. I feel if I can write about the injustices it might promote a better understanding. That is the only reason I write. But it's like being an idiot, because there's a bloody brick wall. Nobody listens. They're too busy telling us who we are and what we are and it's terrible. It's changing, but not much. They've still got to have control of us. We still have a white person in Canberra making decisions and speaking on behalf of Aboriginal people. Charles Perkins should have been our first Aboriginal Minister, but look what they did to him. Down in the hen-house they call Canberra, they're always pecking at one another. I'd like to see Aboriginal people have a voice in government instead of having other people deciding our futures for us.

We need land. This country was not *terra nullius*. That's one dirty big lie, thrown out by the highest court in this land. Captain Cook never discovered this country; there were others that came and went, like the Portuguese and French, but they did not dispossess a people of their land or their dreaming. We're not quite 2 per cent of the total population, and we are on the lowest rung of the social ladder in this country. If people understood what dispossession has done to us, perhaps they would say, 'Hey, here's this most wonderful source of legend, song, and culture that has never been given any acknowledgment in this country. We should be ashamed of ourselves for not giving them a chance and a voice.' It's beginning to happen, but [laughter] it will probably take us another 205 years to pull ourselves out of this shit that's been created for us.

*How strong is your sense of identity, and do you think that your young people will maintain it?*
We've not only got to educate the young ones that don't know nothing—because they're never taught it in the schools—we've also got to educate the thousands that were stolen away and put into homes to train them to be servants to white people. They were forced to turn their back if they saw another Koori person coming up the street. They were not allowed to identify as having any aboriginality. So there's a whole lot of people out there that don't know where the hell they're coming from, because they have been denied their culture and their heritage.

Look, my book is in the HSC this year. Last year was the first time ever in this country that education about Aboriginal people and history was compulsory. Bloody 1992! It's a long way from 1788 to oppress a people. No fair-go there, eh? People either like what I say or they ride me right out of town. Truth is what I am about. Truth. The truth of the matter to promote a better understanding, because there has got to be a coming together of the two cultures, black and white. But on a fair and equal level, not like we are. We're twenty years behind everybody in all the basic human rights' needs of health, housing, education, and employment. It's disgusting. The whole world is watching this country because of this racist attitude.

*Do you think the two cultures will come together as separate cultures, or do you think ultimately they will merge?*

We have always been a separate people; that's our identity. But we have to come together and live together and get on together as equals. Racism is endemic, and it pervades all our institutions whether they be government or privately owned. We are classified as the lowest of the low. It makes me so angry. You know, I wish I were twenty or thirty years younger, I would go round and pop at some people, I would [laughter]. Twenty or thirty years ago, I was battling to raise my kids, working like a man on the fence lines. Sure I was angry, because we never had nothing and we still got nothing.

*What about your parents: were they angry, too? Were they fighters like you?*

No. My dad was a hard worker. He worked for ten or twelve years in one place, and never got into trouble with the law or nothing like that. He was a cricketer; he was captain of the cricket team. We have Aboriginal achievers that could be spoken about in great detail by the media. We own something like 20 to 30 per cent of excellence in sport in this country, and yet look at all the racist flack that we've been copping lately, even with the footballers spitting and calling them names, 'black bastard' and all that. It's disgusting.

My mother ... well, we never got to know our mother, because I was six when she left us, and the other two were four and three. I didn't see her again until we came to Sydney in 1949 when I was fifteen years of age.

*Were you angry with her?*

No. You can have any number of fathers in this world, but you can only have one mother. But the other two sisters never forgave her. I loved my mother; she gave birth to me. I didn't know the name of my mother's mother, and my mother's father was an Italian. My tribal grandmother was raped by an Italian banana plantation owner from Billy Nudgel up in the North coast, so I never knew his name. My grandfather was only one of two Aboriginal cricketers ever to get Sir Donald Bradman out for a duck and Bradman called him a black bastard. Grandfather was going to hit him with the bat [laughter]. He was a stockman, my grandfather. He used to ride on the mission at Box Ridge when I was only a little child, and because I was grumpy and pouting and wouldn't talk, he'd hoist me on top of his seventeen-hand big horse called Kangaroo, and I used to yell out, 'Get me down Poppa, get me down!' [laughter]

*Can you talk about tribal elders and the kind of wisdom they hold?*

We've still got a few of them left; they're not all dead. You see, men and women were the elders. They were all equal, but as the men started to die out, the lore was only recently passed on to the women. We've got one clever one up there, and that's aunty Millie Boyd. She used to keep hold over all our *buthera*, our spirits of the bush. She knows where the blood lines of the whole Bundjalung nation are hidden in the mountains of home. She's said that, because white men have taken too much, she'll take the knowledge to the grave with her. And she's a clever woman. I don't blame her. I don't blame her. Do you understand about the clever people? Well they were likened by that great anthropologist Professor Elkin to the great yogas of Tibet. They had the power to heal. They had the power to kill.

Nimbin Rocks, that's a very sacred place. That's not a woman's country to go to. That's where the clever ones were taught to fly and throw their spirits. The Master is still there, guards that place. That's his spirit that you can feel. It's so sacred that our mob go there, and they sing out and tell the Old One that they're coming. And when they leave they get a twig or branch and brush their footprints off the ground. That's the Master's teaching place.

*And who is the Master?*

The Clever Man. We-un-gali. The white people that have been there have had dreams of a warrior coming with a spear to tell them to get away. It's a very sacred place, same as Mount Lindsay—that's whitefella way of calling it—Mount Lindsay is right on the border between Queensland and New South Wales. You been up that way? The tribal name for that is Julbootherlgoom—see if you can say that! It's the sacred home of the hairy man spirit. I got lost in this place when I was only a little kid, I made a poem up about it; got lost looking for wild fruit, bush lemons and oranges. The only way we got out of that place, we saw a cow with a bell on its neck, hung on to its tail, hit her on the rump with a switch, and she dragged us away.

*As you've got older has your spirituality changed?*
My spirituality is my religion. We've always had that. Yet we had missionaries coming, shoving their doctrines down our throats to change our ways because our traditional ones were classified as heathens and vermin, to be cleared off the face of the earth. But they didn't realise that we had this whole social order before they ever came, and we always knew that we had a good spirit that looked after every living thing. We live in unity with the land; the earth is our mother. We don't come from over the seas. We did not migrate here fifteen thousand years ago when the great ice age lowered the water level and blah, blah, blah, and Papua New Guinea was cut off from the top and Tasmania from the bottom of Australia. We were always here. We come from the earth. In Koori tradition, Aboriginal people were animals and birds and insects before we became humans. Yeah. And the Dreamtime, you know what the Dreamtime is? The Dreamtime is when the spirit forces moved over the land before creation time; like in your Bible when God created heaven and earth, and it took him seven days, and blah, blah, blah. In Koori way, in Dreamtime, the spirit forces moved over the land, and gave it its physical form, the mountains and valleys and trees, and set down the rules for Aboriginal people to live and survive by. We are the world's longest living form of humans.

*The book that was written by Bruce Chatwin—'Songlines'—how did you react?*
I started it and put it down, same as all the other stuff that goes round. Have you read Daisy Bates? I loaned that to my daughter. But you've got a lot of people writing about Aboriginal people when the whole of

the country knows stuff-all and nothin' about us. So you always get the experts portraying their ideas about how we are and what we are on about; but you never hear from our side of the fence. If people want to live in this country and want us to be one, then know this country and know its culture. We are the first people of this land, and that's it in a nutshell. Songlines are secret. They exist, as you see in the paintings where the circles are: it shows where they stopped and camped, and where they moved on. But Aboriginal people made tracks all over this land before white men ever came.

*So tell me how you spend your life now?*

Researching. I've been researching for the past ten years. I've been into everything that's portrayed in the media about Aboriginal people, I've got bags of the stuff. I went to the Historical Society back home to find out all this stuff about grandfather, the cricketer. They had documented evidence about all his family, and they'd got it recorded wrong. It's going to be a big job to restitute the knowledge and fix up all the mistakes that have been made, but we've got to start doing that ourselves. There's a quiet revolution going on, because Aboriginal people are picking up pens and writing their stories, and it's all to promote our people so that we're not twenty to thirty years behind everyone else.

*Has getting older slowed you up?*

You bet it sure has. With all the hard work that I've done over the years, it's a wonder that I'm still standing. But I am, even with a quad stick. And the humour, that's our survival mechanism [laughs]. Oh, dear!

*Are there any advantages in being older?*

Well, I live in this place. I could go and live with my kids who are in the Western suburbs—they are all Westies—but I don't need to be around any more family dramas. I told my kids, 'What goes on from here is mine. I gave life to you'se and helped you'se best I can. You got to get out there and learn to roll with the punches, same as I had to.' But in this place it's ideal, because you're never alone and it's great, it's home. I'm comfortable.

*And the disadvantages of getting older?*

The disadvantages are that I can't get around like I used to for years and years. I've got to have transport everywhere I go. This thing here [waggles quad stick] is only temporary because of the arthritis in my leg. When the summer comes, I reckon I can throw it away. Probably have to get it back by next winter [chuckles].

*Do you feel that you're wiser?*

Oh yes, I'm damn well wiser. But I'm still damned well angry, too. They say anger doesn't solve nothing. It's a negative attitude. But when I research all the injustices that our people have had to put up with in this country, like not getting any acknowledgment for any input in the settling of this land and blah, blah, blah, and how our history has never been taught, it just makes you real angry. And so I try and write—that's my way of dealing with the anger. When I was writing up the massacres of all our people up home on the Evans River, I had all this paper work that I collected up there, and I just had to get up and go away for days and days, do it in bits and pieces. It sickened me that much. They were my extended family in that massacre up there.

It's all over this country, where Koori people's blood has been spilt. There's lots of sacred places that people don't have any respect for. Look at Ayers Rock: they climb all over that. When we went there in 1985 I went and just looked, and it throbbed with power. I couldn't touch it. That's a very sacred place. People have got to learn to respect sacred places if they want the culture—which is the first culture of this land—to ever continue instead of knocking it around and treating it like they do. It's ridiculous. We are the end-result of what dispossession and colonisation has done to us. But there's hope for us, I guess. In Koori way, there's no such thing as coincidence. What happens will happen. Like patterns, it will be, whether you want it or not. It's there. It's a map.

When I went home to research my people after a forty-eight year absence, I thought back to when I was eight years of age and my father took me off that mission to escape a Protection round-up, me and my two sisters. Oh, there's just so much ... I've lost my train of thinking now ... the people that migrated to this country, from all over the world, they don't give away their language or their culture when they sign a piece of paper to become Australian citizens. Yet Aboriginal people were forced to assimilate, forced to give away their language, forced to adopt the ways of the dominant culture, the white bit. No fair-go there. This country knows nothing about that.

*Does your degree of anger ever take a physical form?*

I have many, many headaches. I'm on medication for the cancer, and stuff like that, but I'm still being pushed along. And you know what's pushing me along? The spirit of my people. I tell you, I've never been so bloody motivated in my life [laughs].

*What do you still want to do?*

When my son's probation's is up, we're going to try and get that cultural centre started. But first I want to get a studio here where he can paint, what do you reckon? See, he has to have his own space.

I want to take him home to meet all the tribal ones that he's been painting though photographs while he was in jail. There's two books I want to go along with, but I've got to slow up because I am tired. After all the sorrows and sadness that I've been writing, I've got a book of Koori humour called *Only Gammon*. 'Only Gammon' in urban Koori slang means 'not real.' I'm going to be interviewing Koori people for their favourite stereotyped jokes—the ones we make up that hit back at the system that stereotyped us all our lives.

*Do you worry about running out of time?*

The body mightn't be able to get around as fast as I used to, but as long as the old brain is ticking over I want to write my son's book about jail. He did six years' jail for something he never did. But because he was the eldest of three teenagers, police had to have a conviction and that was it. Gone! Same as our Aboriginal boys with deaths in custody. Our people are being brutalised. You ask any Koori, and still they're dying. They're dying for minor things, and what it says is that our people are being brutalised by the disreputable jail system in this country. They put it down to suicide, and say 'cultural circumstances'. There were some, but there was also a lot of cover-ups. They gave a thirty-million grant for an inquiry into that and yet that thirty million never went into helping the families of those that died. It went to the big-shot lawyers on the case. There's laws good for the white man but never for the black.

*How many of your children died—you had nine?*

Three.

*Is that grief still with you?*

No. My children are gone. They're in the spirit world.

*What does that mean?*

We believe in reincarnation. Aboriginal way, we come back as a totem. I'm a Willie Wagtail, that's my totem messenger bird; it talks to me now when things are going to happen. If you read my book, you'll understand. I explain it in great detail.

*Are you scared of dying?*

No. Everything that lives and breathes is born to die. We're not immortal, none of us. We're flesh, and we go back into the earth where we come from, the earth that's nurtured us all our lives. We go back into our mother's arms.

*Do you ever get lonely?*

No. Because in this place you don't get a chance to get lonely. We've got boys and girls yarning, the elder ones. But the boys sit at one table and the girls at the other, we give them cheek. I had four goes at finding that elusive thing called love. I lived with four men, two Koories and two Gubbs. I married a Gubb, so I know what it's like from both sides of the fence. But, no, all I ever wanted was a working man, and all I ever ended up with was the bums. The kids used to say to me,' Mum, don't talk about our dads like that! ' But I've been on my own for a good few years. I couldn't be bothered having a man telling me what to do. I know where I am going and what to do. I enjoy my life, what I've got.

I'm not much of a social person like I used to be. I don't drink or smoke any more, and I can't go to hear bands in hotels like I used to, because the cigarette smoke kills me. And my kids say to me, 'Mum, you can't beat a reformed drunk or a reformed person.' But my kids are the most important thing that I've ever had. I've got a good rapport with the whole lot of them. I've got twenty-one grandchildren, last count. Thank goodness they don't come and visit me all at the one time, because we'd need a football field. I write about my kids all the time, because I've got an unlimited source of Aboriginal achievement, comedy, drama—the whole bit.

*Do you want to die at home?*

Yeah, where I come from. But my kids are buried here, so's my father and my mother. They should have been buried back up home, but that was the way it's meant to be. My grandfather's buried on the mission, so's my aunty Phyllis. They've still got a segregated cemetery there. Home for me is not the mission where I was born; it's got so many sad memories for me. Home is a little town called Bonalbo. That's where we went to school; we went to Sunday School, we went to little concerts with my sisters—no racism there. We were the only Koories in the township. I can still go back and walk into that pub where I worked as a chamber maid emptying out the jerry pots—and as soon as they see me coming, they gave me heaps. They yell, 'Look, there she is coming, our famous author. Ruby's home!'

*How would you like to be remembered?*

As a mother, grandmother, a fighter for human rights and social justice for my people. That's how I'd like to be remembered. That's what I do.

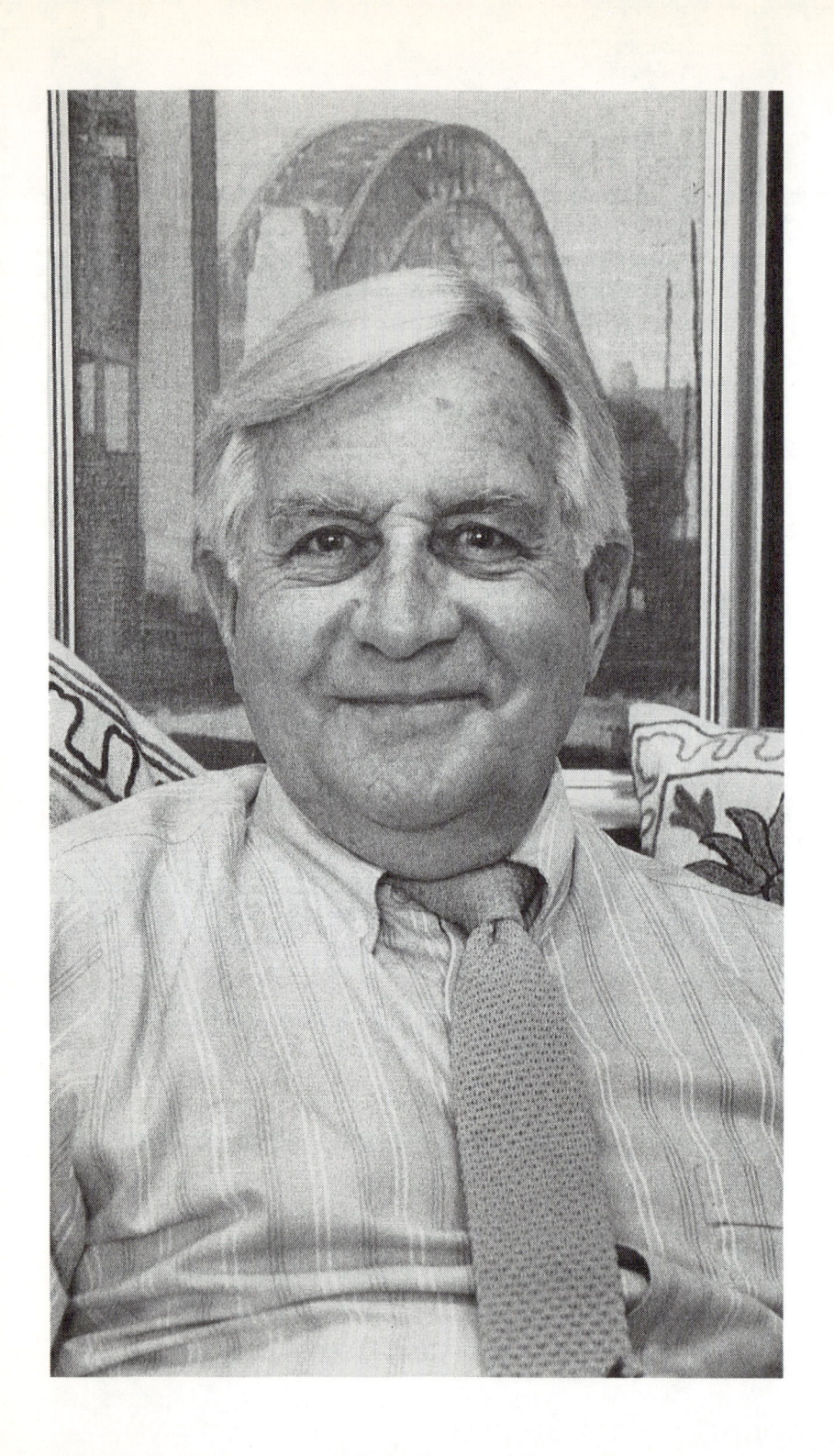

# John Kingsmill
*In place*

John Kingsmill is a writer, raconteur, and social historian who has done much to make an earlier era of Sydney come vividly alive. His first two books, *The Innocent* and *Australia Street*, were about Australia in the 1920s and 1930s—in particular, about his own boyhood, growing up in Sydney's Bondi. His third book (1994), is called *No Hero*, and recounts his experiences in the second world war.

Kingsmill was born in Sydney in September 1920, and talks movingly about his childhood and how this relates to his present experiences as a man in his seventies. He comes from a family of battlers, left school at fifteen, eventually gained accreditation as an accountant, had a brief spell as a professional actor, and somewhere along the way founded a rehabilitation organisation for people who were mentally ill. At the age of forty-two he began a new and successful career as an advertising copywriter.

John Kingsmill retired in 1981, taught himself to paint, and began writing his books. He lives in a quiet, comfortable Sydney apartment, full of books and pictures. He loves beaches, good music, art, books and conversation, and says he admires a survivor.

My grandparents were an enormous factor in our lives as children. My grandmother was a tremendously strong little lady with white hair piled up on top of her head and little round glasses. She was the centre of the family. Not that she exerted power over the family in a matriarchal way but she was a bank of love that we used to draw on. She'd been through very hard times. The great depression of the 1890s in Australia tipped them out of the house that they had rented in Paddington. Possessions were taken away from people who owed rent. They were left with nothing—pots and pans and a couple of mattresses. And so because she had been through all this, and survived with a tremendous sense of humour, my grandmother became a rock-like figure. This rubbed off on all of us—not only the enormous affection we had for her, and the big store of memories, but I think she taught us a lesson of survival and the importance of a sense of humour. She was a great laugher, and we were all laughers as a result. Even in hard times we laugh. It must look very crazy to other people, but it is a sort of release and a defiance of bad times.

The other old people beyond gran and our grandfather, who was a dear old Scotsman, were the old people we saw around us. They were all important to us at Bondi. We were taught to respect age, and to demonstrate that respect by getting out of their way if they were walking on the footpath, or by offering them a seat, or deferring to them if they were getting on to a tram or were in a shop. So you became very conscious of people being old.

It was a long, long time before you realised that people you loved—your older relatives and people who lived close by—were starting to die. And the great shock of this made me realise that old people were precious in the sense that they weren't going to be with us all that long. And so what you had to learn from them, and what you were supposed to give to them, could not be overlooked. It had to be observed in the sense of the observation of religious feasts—an observation of the fact of old people not being here very long.

**So the death of your grandmother must have been very traumatic for you?**

Yes, it was. I don't think our family ever got over it. They still talk about the old lady, and when she went it was a disaster for the family. Having learned from her how to survive, we had to mend ourselves and be content with the memory of the woman. She was to us a great person. When they go, you think you're never going to get over it, that it's the end of the world. It's not. If they have been truly great, they have left something behind to help you survive.

*What qualities do you think she gave you?*
A tremendous sense of humour and fun. I get into trouble sometimes. My grandmother was down to earth, and even though I've done my best to be a gentleman all my life, I am fundamentally very earthy and will roar with laughter at earthiness. I like it.

*Reading your book,* The Innocent, *I had a sense of a very rich childhood, full of people and experiences. Do your brothers and sisters feel the same way?*
I wish I could say yes. I think one or two of them do. We've all grown out of it, of course, and I don't know that we all see the good there was in the old days. Some do, some less so. Maybe we dream too much about these times, and have been too much under their spell. I wouldn't want to lose that. It's too precious to me; it's part of me.

*In the biographical notes to one of your books it says that you admire a survivor. Do you see your mother in the same terms?*
Even more so, because my mother went through that same Depression of the 1890s when she was a young girl. By then, there were three or four children, and she was the eldest—what I guess the Russians would call Little Mother in the family. The First World War came, and then she got married in 1918 and had a big family. There were six of us: five boys then a girl. I'm the eldest. Almost simultaneously with the arrival of the sixth child, the second Depression came—the 1920 crash—and my father went out of business almost immediately. Bankrupt. Which sparked off his alcoholism. There were minor episodes during the 1920s, and long episodes on and off through the 1930s when I was at school.

We didn't know about alcoholism in those days, you see. We thought he was a 'drunk', and he wasn't a drunk at all. He was an alcoholic, a sick man, and we didn't know that for many, many years afterwards. So that was immensely painful. I don't think I thought about much else, except when I was at the movies, or surfing, or dancing. These were antidotes, but they were momentary. The fundamental basis of my life had everything to do with the awful struggle in our house to survive poverty and to survive the chaos.

*You use the word 'chaos'. Yet what comes through in your writing is that yours was a family with a lot of ritual: you talk about the ritual of Christmas and so on. Is that important to you now?*

No. When my mother died ten years ago, Christmas ended for me. It's an annual crisis. If I want to I can go to my brother's place for Christmas; but I don't want to, because she's not there. My brother's children are perfectly good young people: they're married; they've got partners and children, and so on; but it's a completely different scene, and I'm not part of it.

*Why do you think this is?*

I have stood still and they have gone on. I have stayed on the same road that was laid down for me by my mother and my grandmother, and by me taking it up and making variations, and becoming different from my family. Once I physically moved away from my family, I pursued mental and taste pursuits and the dictates of my own mind. I didn't have to think what they thought. I became interested in theatre and good music and so on, and in meeting people—nothing to do with my family life at all. I became independent of my family. I still see them from time to time, but it's like taking a journey to visit another country, the old country. So, Christmas I find very painful. I think most single people do. You're supposed to be sitting down with loved ones and spending the whole middle of the day with them. I find that a bit hard, because when you spend most of your time alone, being with a crowd of other people for longer than three or four hours, it finally becomes like a cage, and I have to get away and be by myself for a while. That's not pathological. I've learned to enjoy my own company.

*I wonder whether that is a characteristic of getting older—that you do need more quiet, more space?*

I think I've always been like that. Quiet and space are enormously important to me. I hate loud noise, unless its a symphony orchestra in full cry, which I love. And I love the roar of a crowd, like at a football match—but I'm part of that, I'm helping to make that noise. A very loud argument in the street will upset me. If I hear people abusing each other, I find that deeply disturbing. The crash of something falling and breaking. Also, the confinement of space. I can happily sit in a crowded theatre but, given a choice, I will sit where there are empty seats around me. I found it very difficult to make friends when I was a kid. I did have *some* friends, but no longstanding friendships compared with my gregarious brothers. I had a life which could be described almost as lonely.

*And now?*
I'm going through a strange phase now. It makes me sad to think that, although about twenty or thirty years ago I ran into a period in my life in which I was making lots of friends and being popular, that has almost totally disappeared. Now I just occasionally get an invitation or have people here. I used to be able to sit down preparing an invitation list and, without even thinking, write down twenty names of people I liked very much, people I felt I *had* to ask. Now, if I get to ten I am starting to scratch.

*Why do you think this has happened?*
I think that people have lost interest in me because I'm no longer such good company. I used to love making people laugh, and still would if I felt able to. People love to laugh; they don't want to have a sour-puss around. I think what happened to me in the last twenty years is what's happened to a lot of people of my age. They've become deeply conscious of the rapid change in their surroundings, in the community, in politics. I have greater respect now for the man who wrote *Future Shock* than I did then. I know what he's talking about—revolution, the rapidity of change especially in tastes and manners and attitudes, sex and drugs and rock & roll. Unless you moved along with it you'd be left far, far behind.

And so I no longer understand people of forty. I would love to have friends of forty. They would stimulate me enormously, and I might have something to offer them by way of mental stimulation. I don't know, because I simply don't know anybody of forty. I hardly know anyone of fifty. Most of the people I see are comparatively new friends, and they are all my age or older than I am.

*But what about your contemporaries who were your friends? What's happened to them?*
Some of them have died, and many of them have moved away. This is an exploding city. And because I don't drive, I find it just that much more difficult to get about—changing buses, changing trains. It's just one more barrier. But also those people belonged to a rather more

fun-loving period of my life; and I've come out of that, I'm sad to say, because I enjoyed it. We've moved apart.

*So what kind of a life are you in now?*
My mood is connected with my writing. I was a very serious boy and a shy boy, and the shy, serious boy has emerged again as an old man.

*That's interesting, because I've often wondered whether we do revert to the kind of people we were as children.*
I think that what's happening with me proves that the leopard doesn't change its spots. All these wonderful cliches that we were taught never to use, why not use them if they work? I think I'm reverting to nature. I might turn into a little baby one day.

*Are you lonely?*
Yes. I would never have admitted that a few years ago. But, yes, I am lonely. I love conversation, as you can tell from this. But there are *very* few people to talk to in my life, to talk to like this. So what I try to do is to ask somebody here; usually one, sometimes two people, and we just sit and talk over a drink or a dish of tea. Or I visit them and the same thing happens.

*Okay, so living like this, a much more solitary life than before, what other effects does it have on you? For example, do you find yourself thinking of your health much more than before?*
I do think of my health much more than I used to. I know that hypochondria is based on no fact at all. I'm not sick. I've got the usual aches and pains. I've had arthritis on and off since I was about thirty-five—that's a very long time. I think that my constitution and state of health, thank God, I derive from my mother, because she was an abundantly healthy woman. But she did have very bad arthritis, and mine is getting slowly worse. I've got it under control with a tablet that I take. The thing that upsets me most of all is that it's stopped me from taking my long walks. I used to go for five-kilometre walks through Centennial Park, and in the summer-time up and down the water's edge at Bondi Beach several times, five days a week. And that kept me healthy, kept my weight down! Well, because the arthritis has struck me in the feet, specially my right foot, I've had to cut way back for the time being. There are one or two other little things which are very

minor and transitory, but I shouldn't kick against that because I don't see that at seventy-two I should expect to feel as healthy as I did when I was twenty-two. I had enormously good health. We all did. We were given that, if we were given nothing else. Abundant good health. Vigorous good health. And we used it to the limit. The passing of that is part of the feeling of regret about being old.

*Are there other regrets?*

The loss of appearance. I'm vain enough to think that I might have been quite good looking once, and I think sometimes the reason why I'm not invited out as much as I used to be is that nobody wants to see an old man walk in. That's what I am, and that's what I look like. I don't think I'm an old man in my mind; in fact I'm damned sure I'm not, except that social occasions are for people to look their best, and it's very hard for me to manage that now, in my mind. My best is past.

*But is that an attitude of our times, because you talked about how in your childhood people respected old age? Is it harder now to be old?*

I don't think it would be in wiser cultures like the Chinese and other cultures which revere the old. But I don't think they have cocktail parties!

*You could have dish-of-tea parties.*

Or exchange-of-flower parties. It would be lovely, wouldn't it! Our culture increasingly worships youth. We can see it all the time. Everyone who appears on television looks like a child, or young at least; and even those who aren't young have been got up to look young and beautiful. Going to the beach, which was an enormous part of my life when I was young, has become an embarrassment because of what I now look like in speedos. I try to avoid the beach at the weekends, when the beach belongs to the young. The sight of that is so poignant to me; I feel out of place. I don't like feeling out of place. I like to feel *in* place. When I go to a symphony concert I am inconspicuous: I am dressed properly, I observe concert manners, I have my own opinions about whether the performance is good or not, but I behave impeccably as a member of that audience. I am in place.

*Maybe we could all go down to the beach in togas.*

That would be beautiful. I can remember when I was little, men wore dressing gowns to the beach, and women wore kimonos. They were dressed up to be on the beach.

*Have you ever thought of having a face lift?*

Never. No, no, no [laughs]. I don't want to do anything cosmetic apart from the usual after-shave things. No, I would hate myself for that. If you're in show business and your face is your fortune, you have to do things like that. But if you're not in show business and you're doing it out of vanity, I think it's pathetic.

*Was there a stage at which you first realised you were getting older?*

Yes. I had the most awful awareness of it one day, and I thought, 'How long has this been going on? Have I caught up with myself at last?' But it might also have been that I have such an acute perception of myself that I caught it, not the instant it happened, but early on.

*Has getting older affected your relationships? Have you always been on your own or have you had partners?*

Very briefly, partners early on. But that ended many years ago, and I never tried again; it was all too painful when it ended. And so I fell back on myself. I had friends instead of partners, and I told myself that I was not the type to spend a life with another person. I don't know if that's true or not, because I'd never tried to live with someone else—maybe a reaction to my chaotic childhood. For a while I *shared* a flat, perhaps once or twice, and we got on quite well, had a lot of laughs; but I was very glad to get a place of my own. I knew that I was going to be lonely in this place of my own, but it was all mine.

There were times when I came through the front door, and closed it, when I was glad about that. I could shut out the rest of the world with all its sweetness gone, and all its increasing dangers—I'm talking about the mugging and thuggery, and all that menacing atmosphere in the streets. I think the world has become uglier in the last twenty or thirty years. People no longer look nice. There are so many people who look positively dangerous, strange, and freakish. They probably aren't all dangerous at all. They are dressing in the fashion of the day, like gipsies—ragged, unkempt, all that unwashed hair, and earrings, and grubbiness. Now I regard that as abnormal. But I've stopped seeing it.

When that first erupted around 1970 and seemed to take over society,

I wasn't willing to accept what I thought was madness. So when I got into my flat and shut the door, that was my little kingdom where I called all the shots. If I wanted to put Mozart on, I put Mozart on. If I wanted to work, I worked. If I wanted to talk to myself silently in my mind, which I think I do practically all the time—I think we all do—then I could do that, untroubled, uninfluenced by people whose notions of life are so different from mine. So, yes, I've been left behind by rapidly changing times.

*I have a sense that we probably measure our lives in peaks and troughs—we forget the bits in the middle unless we're actually being very introspective—so what are the peaks and troughs in your life?*

Youthful things first, frivolous things, because they're the best. I became a very good body-surfer. Even though I was never a strong swimmer, I could really catch the shoots. Apart from being at least as good as the others, the very physical act of riding a wave before it broke and *as* it breaks, and riding it to the beach, is one of the most beautiful things that man can possibly do, because it so closely connects with nature. No board, just the body and the wave. Beautiful. I miss it!

When I learned that I could dance, and dance extremely well, and had a tremendous sense of rhythm, that went on for years and years. I was one of the little wave of young dancers who broke down the barriers to jitterbugging. I'm talking about the 1930s in the Eastern Suburbs where I became an expert 'free dancer'. A jitterbug!

Getting to Sydney High School was a great triumph for me, because the selective school system was quite new in 1933, and to be chosen on merit was a real peak in my life. It was one of the great thrills of my mother's life when she took me there on the first day of the school year. It's in my book, *The Innocent*. But it also was a day of personal tragedy for me, because I was put into the wrong course of study. I should have been put in the classics course; but there was no advice, no aptitude testing, nothing. In my ignorance I went and sat with the boys who were going to do commercial subjects. That changed my life —such a small thing that led to my becoming an accountant. I never wanted to.

Surviving the war was a great release, an explosion of joy when the war ended. I didn't want to go to war, but I had to go. That's what my new book is about. It's called *A Slow-footed Volunteer*. Four years of my young life gone, but I survived, thank God.

I became an actor, briefly, and I'll write a book about that if God spares me (I've already begun it). It was always a thrill to go out on to the stage and give a performance that was applauded, however mediocre that performance might have been. I was sometimes far better than mediocre, I believe, but I gave it up and went back to accountancy.

My life in the 1950s, when I was in my thirties, became madly complicated—highs and lows all jumbled up. For reasons I won't go into here, I became involved in a small social club for the patients at Callan Park Mental Hospital. These were very bad times in the mental health field: appalling conditions, appalling administration, major political scandals, a royal commission. We set up a formal body, the Psychiatric Rehabilitation Association (PRA), and I very soon became its chairman and its prime mover. I worked day and night at it, learning as I went. I had no experience in charity work, in public life, in public speaking; but there I was bringing people into what was called 'an unpopular cause.' I had to overcome official obstruction and public indifference, but we got there finally. In my five years as leader we acquired clubs and premises, and a small bank account, and a fund-raiser. We had a viable community service. I stood down as chairman and found myself, aged forty, with no job, no prospects, and had to start all over again. I should never have done it. But if I hadn't, who would have done it? I wonder who, if anybody, remembers what I did.

In 1957, I took up public speaking and became not only a first-rate speaker in a very short time but I was elected club critic evaluating the speeches of men twenty years my senior—lawyers, and so forth—and being applauded for that. I became deeply respected, perhaps for the first time in my life. This was a talent I'd secretly known about for many many years, but was too shy to reveal. It was better than acting. When you are a public speaker you write your own material; you are the playwright *and* actor. And when you are at all good at it, it's a tremendous personal achievement. The applause is deeply satisfying. I no longer pursue this. It's over.

Just after I turned forty, I decided I couldn't make a life career of accountancy. So I switched to advertising. I became a copywriter, again without any experience whatsoever. I found I had a natural bent for it. I survived the rat-race, and went on to be an associate creative director (a meaningless title) in Australia's biggest advertising agency. I had begun much too late to be regarded as executive material, so I spent my days in a back room, writing good scripts for someone else to present.

I don't think management ever knew what I did for the agency bank account.

*Looking ahead, are there experiences you would still like to have?*

The experience of feeling well, and being vigorous and independent, physically, mentally and emotionally, is enormously important to me. I've been lucky so far. I want to achieve—this will sound pompous, forgive me—a body of work by the time I'm ready to stop writing, and I don't think I ever will stop. I'd like to achieve, say, six books that people love and respect, and sometimes being asked to speak. I occasionally go down to the University of Wollongong. The English department there took up my book, *The Innocent*, and put it in the Australian autobiography course. I have also spoken to more mature academic audiences, again on autobiography. Now I'm a boy who left school at fifteen. Yet I am not looking upon that as a triumph; I am looking on that as recognition. I would like one or two of my books to go into the HSC (Higher School Certificate) course. It's not the money. The reason I would like to think that one or two of my books eventually become subjects of study is because then I would leave something behind. That's why I am writing—to leave something behind.

*If a young person came to you now and asked for counsel on how to live their life, what might you say to them?*

It starts with what my mother used to say: be good, behave yourself, never let yourself down. Never tell lies, unless you're in something like a life-threatening situation. Never cheat. Work hard. Always be kind if you have the opportunity to be kind. Be helpful where you can. Think before you speak, particularly if you are angry. Be loving. Never hesitate to tell someone you love them if you love them, because they might not always be around for you to tell them, and they need to know. If you believe strongly in something, say it. Be brave enough to be in opposition. Be brave enough to be the only person who thinks as you do, because if you speak out you might discover other people who think as you do; if you don't speak out, all of the people of your turn of mind could remain silent and be swept away into the garbage bin, and would deserve it.

Above all, to thine own self be true. Discover who you are and what you are; it might not be what the world expects you to be, but you still have to be that person, and you must be honest about it. If you are not honest to yourself, you are living a lie. Beyond all of that, enjoy life. You are only young once. Remain fresh, ready to take up new ideas, to discover new things in yourself. You must be prepared to take these journeys in order to live life to the fullest. The worst thing that could happen to anyone is to stay in the same circle of people from the beginning of your life to the end. We should spread the net very widely, and discover what an amazing array of people there is in the world. We could live to be thousands of years old, and never plumb the depths of that reservoir.

*It is interesting hearing you talk, because there seems to be a paradox between the John Kingsmill who wants to go out and ask questions, and wants experiences, and is receptive and perceptive; and the other one who comes back, and shuts the door, and needs solitude.*

That's part of being shy. Locked inside the shy person is an extrovert; and inside that extrovert, a shy person. So I'm both. But always this very strong awareness of the things that make me different from other people. I don't regard myself as average, except perhaps physically. The best way to be immediately accepted everywhere is to be like everybody else. I am not like everybody else, and I revel in that. I am glad. It has made me a loner. I would rather have that than be somebody wearing a white hat that says *Edgecliff* and playing bowls. I know there are splendid people playing bowls right now, even though its raining, but I couldn't bear it for myself. I would rather just sit here and write, or just sit and think.

*John, does God have any meaning for you?*

Oh, yes. My mother made me believe in God by teaching me the Lord's Prayer when I was very young. I don't think a night has gone by in my life when I haven't ended my day, after I have turned the light out, by saying the Lord's Prayer. She also taught me to say prayers afterwards for all of my family; and it was a big family, so that besides my parents, grandparents, and brothers and sister, there was a long string of names to be named afterwards.

God is a presence in my life because I can't bear the thought that there is no power of that kind which we call God. I cannot bear the thought that our lives consist of nothing but being born, growing, declining, and dying. I think that there is a soul in each of us, and that soul is the expression of God in this body. So I pray. Take, for instance,

God forbid, a plane accident. I think that most people would, in their own particular ways, pray or turn to God. That is because we have built into our minds an awareness that we really are helpless creatures. We need to have some feeling that there is a power that—if it can't save us—will receive us and take us out of that disaster into something which is completely unknown. We don't know what it is, but the hope is that there is something beyond the chaos and the unsolved problems of our lives.

Apart from that, I find the notion of God very beautiful because it lifts me above the dirt, and it gives me a feeling that I am reaching out into an element which *might* be a figment of my mind—but why is it there, why do I think there is a God? And if I think there *is* a God, then there is a God. There is a God of some kind in all cultures; man had a need of God. But that's a negative way of looking at it. I have a much more positive view of God. I think that God as a word comes from the word 'good.' I think that God and good are words—and ideas—that are related, and have always had a connection, as have the words evil and devil. I think we have mixed in us capacities which would horrify us if we knew what we were capable of, and that the element of God is the thing that balances good and evil in us. Each man is capable of evil, but each man is capable of resisting evil. And if that's all God is, he has kept us going.

*Are you frightened of dying?*
If it is going to be swift and comparatively painless—and these days they know how to get rid of pain—and certainly not agonisingly prolonged, as my poor mother's death was, then I'm not afraid. I'd like to know that my house was in order, that my papers were right, that I had a good will, and that I didn't leave problems behind. If I can do that, leave nothing unresolved, no debts, leave a decent amount of money to people who will need it—fundamentally, my family—then, no, I am not afraid.

*What would you like people to say about you?*
'He was a good man. I loved him. I'll miss him. He made my life better. I owe him a great deal. I've got his books to read. I remember how much we used to laugh. He was intelligent. I enjoyed talking to him. He was kind.'

That's all.

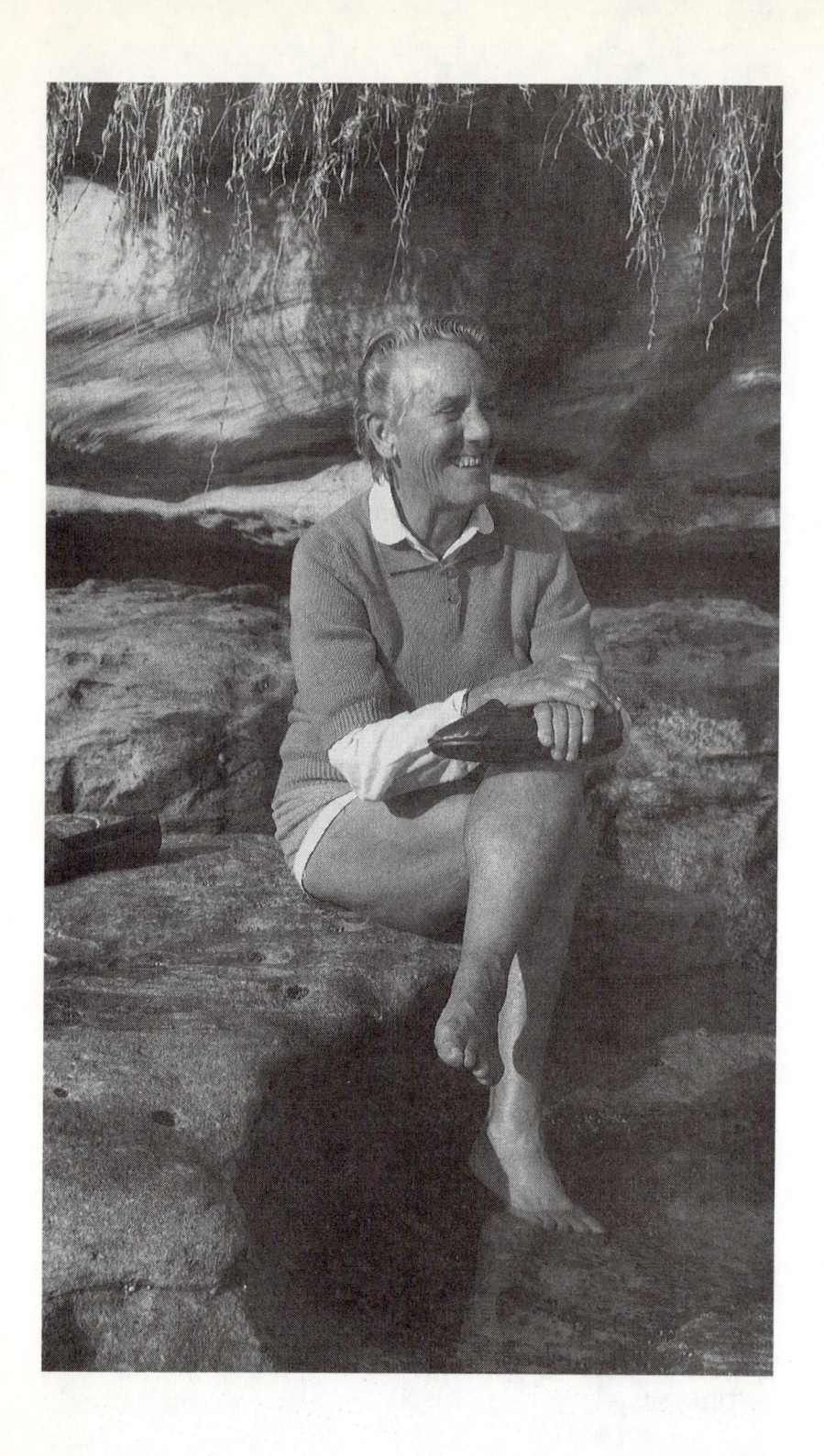

# Freda Brown
## *My valuable wrinkles*

Freda Brown was born in Sydney in June 1919. For many years she was president of the Union of Australian Women, the Women's International Democratic Federation, and vice-president of the World Peace Council. Now, she is involved in activities concerned with ageing, such as a senior media network and a national action plan for dementia care. She says that it all sounds a mouthful, 'but in fact I'm really a token oldie on them.'

In fact, it is impossible ever to conceive of Freda Brown being any kind of token: her views are strong, well-argued, and direct. She believes that old age can be a rewarding time but, like most things, it needs preparation and education. When her journalist husband, Bill, developed Alzheimer's disease, she nursed him for four years until his death in 1992; both she and Bill featured in a moving documentary on Alzheimer's, *You must Remember This*.

Freda has one daughter and three grandchildren, walks vigorously along Bondi Beach where she has lived for many years, and has a house full of books, files, grandchildren's toys, and memorabilia.

My father was a sign-writer until I was about ten. You know, we were an ordinary working-class family. But then came unemployment, and that terrible period is still clear in my mind. At first, like a lot of people, my father was very proud, and he wouldn't get the dole or relief. I remember when I was very young being sent to get some butter from my uncle who worked in Newtown markets. He just said 'Stand over there!' I must have stood for half an hour, thinking to myself, 'I'd rather we didn't have butter than have to do this.' Mum used to roll up newspapers, and the Chinese would take your roll of newspaper and give you vegetables. So my childhood was very hard. But I never doubted the love of my mum, dad and my two little brothers, no matter how poor we were.

*Do you look back on that childhood as a happy time?*

Mixed, mixed. There was insecurity because of being so poor, but also much that was happy. I can remember I used to take my brothers to the pictures; it was sixpence each, so I used to put one brother on my back and get the other one to look small. Many times we got in for one sixpence and then we could buy lollies!

We'd go down to the park and play cricket with dad and the two boys. It's interesting to look at some of the photos: we look quite ragged [laughs]. You used to get dole clothes, but then everyone knew you were on the dole. So I preferred ragged clothes. I also got clothes from wealthy relatives. When I was going to school I'd stuff newspaper in the soles of my shoes because I had holes in them, and then put on polish. Dad came out while I was doing it, and he said, 'What are you doing?' I said, 'I've got a hole in my shoe.' I can remember I looked up, and for the first time realised he was crying.

*Did he get work eventually?*

Well, he set up his own sign-writer's business and I worked with him for a while as a sign-writer. That was the first time I came into public notice because it was bit unusual. They came out and took a photo of me sitting on the ladder painting signs, with a caption 'First Woman Sign-writer.'

*Did you have old people in your life then? Grandparents?*

Only grandmothers. Girls at school used to talk about their grandfathers, and I always wished I had a grandfather. I was quite fond of both of my grandmothers, and my mothers' mother died in our house. I remember I went into the room and saw my grandmother dead. It was an important experience. I think we need to get away from all these terms like 'passed away'. We won't say 'dead!'. We must accept age and death, and not be frightened of it. Life is limited, and all living things come and go.

*Do you remember going into your grandmother's room when she was dead?*
Yes. When I close my eyes it's like a photo. It was a little back bedroom where my uncle also died. That was the room that I was then able to have, but I never felt fear because people had died in it. I can see Grandma very clearly. There she was. She was a very little thing with white hair and she'd always had the bun. But now it was let down and her hair was over her shoulders. She looked very peaceful. There was no fear. I was interested to see it and to see her.

When Bill died, my daughter Lee and I were with him, and then Lee wanted the children to see him so we went out to the mortuary. I feel that was a mistake, because to look at a person when they've just died is different to seeing them cold quite a few days later. Something had happened. It wasn't Bill; he wasn't there at all. We all just sat around and I kissed him. Now I wish I'd stayed longer with him immediately after he died. Then there is still part of them there; but when it's a few days later, and you touch the body, it's ice-cold. I wasn't happy about that.

*Going back to your childhood, what was school like for you?*
Well, because we were very poor, everything was a struggle—to get a uniform, to get books, etc. But still I think I was happy. I enjoyed school.

*Did you have a clear idea of what you wanted to do when you left school?*
No, tragically I didn't, because of this financial problem. The boys were coming up, and so I left. It was interesting how I came to leave. I didn't have a scholarship to go to university, which was my only hope of going, and of course we didn't have any money. So I went back to repeat another year, and by pure chance we learned about the New Theatre. It was called 'Art as a Weapon'. They put on plays about the

working class. Clifford Odets wrote 'Till the Day I Die' and it was banned. It was a wonderful play about the horrors of the Nazis coming to power in Germany. I was so taken with it, I went home to dad and said I would like to leave. And I worked with the theatre for a period; I acted and did a bit of production.

*Was yours a political household?*

Oh, very much so. My father was in the no-conscription campaign of the first world war. He had been jailed for his no-conscription activity. So he was very political.

*And your mother?*

Not at all. In fact, I think she resented it. Dad was always out at meetings, etc, but that was my model from an early age. When dad got over that first terrible hump of shame, then he quickly joined what was called the UWM, the Unemployed Workers Movement. They met at our house. He used to conduct educational programs because, though he wasn't a university man, he was really very learned. He used to teach people about anthropology and read Shakespeare to them. So that was good, because it gave me a love of Shakespeare.

*After the New Theatre, what happened?*

Bill, my future husband, came into the theatre to write. He wrote a lot of plays. Some people think that street theatre is a recent development, but we used to put theatre on in the back of lorries —frequently for the Labor Party. I can remember one well, 'Headlines of the Week'. There were three of us, and we had a stand which we would flick over and you'd see the headlines— the threat of war and what was happening in Germany. And then we got married. For a short while I worked as a journalist, and then stood for parliament a whole number of times as a communist.

Bill was working on the *Mirror* at the time, and I'd stood for the Senate, and they used to declare it on the street. All the candidates were invited, the defeated as well as the successful, so we stood around and then each one was given the right to speak. Of course, being a communist you always took the opportunity to speak, even if no-one was there. So I got up and held forth, and Bill came with a few other journalists. I ran after him, and he just said, 'This is my wife.' The men looked at me in horror and walked away. Bill stood there laughing and said, 'We were walking down the street and they said, "God, fancy being married to that last speaker!" At that moment you run up and I say, 'Meet my wife.' [laughter]

*Did you both become members of the Communist Party together?*
Oh no, I recruited him [laughter].

*So what led you into membership of the party?*
Well, I suppose it was dad and my training and seeing the injustice. When I left school, for instance, I just couldn't get a job. I remember walking into town and standing in a queue at a chocolate shop, for an hour. Why they couldn't just select someone, I don't know. And then I had to walk home to Erskinville. If there is misery, people latch on to it to make money out of it; and in those days the unemployed were very much exploited. There was an ad for young women and all the things they offered; but when you went in, it was an agency and you had to pay ten shillings to register, ten shillings to have your photograph taken, and so on. There was never any offer of a job. These kind of injustices stirred me up. And the threat of war, that was a big thing in our youth—the horror of the First World War and the threat of the Second World War. That had an enormous effect on me.

*What happened when war began?*
Bill joined the army and I used to go around the countryside speaking to raise money for government war loans. Then later on I went into the Union of Australian Women—first it was the New Housewives. There were all kinds of campaigns by women, different kinds of campaigns to what they have today, but they attracted me to the women's movement and that's where I worked after that.

*In those early days, what were you working towards?*
There was rationing, high prices, the need for housing and, all the time, women's rights, and particularly equal pay and child care—they played a very big part in the women's movement in those days.

*How do you feel about what's happening now?*
In spite of the 1975 International Women's' Year and the growth of the women's movement, I feel that to some extent we have gone backwards. In winning equality, women now carry the burden of earning

the living and caring for the home. There has been some change—some young men participate more—but I still feel women have terrible problems. Cruelty against women is very worrying to me. We have not really advanced in positions of power. We are nowhere near equality. Women's liberation has achieved a great deal, but I do have some reservations about it. I feel that they were too anti-men. I think some men have made a very big contribution to women's fight for equality, but some men don't know where they are going and don't know what their place in society is. When you raise this with some women they will say, 'We've suffered. Let them suffer.' I don't see it like that. I would like men and women to work together for better relationships and a better world.

*When you talked just then about violence towards women—that's not something that's new, though.*

It was hidden. Now, thank God, it's out in the open. Of course it took place. I remember just in our family, my aunty—her husband, he throttled her. He used to thrash all the children. Her eldest son learned to box, and came home one night and belted him, and said, 'Next time you touch mum or the kids I'll kill you.'

*As you have got older do you think you have become wiser?*

Yes. I have my own personal campaign at the moment, and that is to change the image of 'old.' I get so sad when old people say, 'I'm not old.' I say, 'You are old, I'm old, and there is nothing wrong with being old.' In pre-literate society I doubt if people would have denied being old. Elders were respected for the value of their learning and knowledge. Today, people are afraid of being old, but you shouldn't be afraid. Look how much money is spent on the collagen or whatever they pump into you, so you won't have wrinkles. I say to my grandchildren, 'See my wrinkles, I've earned every one of them. And those grey hairs, I've earned every one of them. You haven't got them, have you? You haven't earned them yet; you've got to work hard before you'll have those very valuable wrinkles and grey hair!'

That may sound a bit silly, but I just feel that you've got to get across the idea that there is nothing to be ashamed of. All right, so you creak. And there are certain complaints that come with age. So, there were certain complaints that came with childhood. It's another period, and people need to see that. As far as I'm concerned, I don't know that

I am any wiser; but I'm more tolerant, and I think that's important.

*Do you think that people are more resistant now to getting old, more inclined to cloak it in euphemisms than when you were growing up?*

Yes, because we have made it so much a young person's world, particularly the media. When do you see the old on the media? When do you see the old on television? It's all young, it's all slim. I think that's very sad because, as I say, everyone will get old. Maurice Chevalier said it beautifully: 'There is only one alternative, and it's not a very nice one.' If you live long enough, you reach old age; and every age has its value. Don't decry grey hairs and wrinkles. Realise that they are part of life. The one thing I regret and resent about getting old is losing the people I love. That is terrible. Apart from that, even with all the creaks, I don't object to it.

*Yet in talking to people, this is the part that they seem to mind the most: the fact that they start to become physically frailer, and that they ache. But you are able to accept that?*

Well, I do something about it. I do yoga twice a week. I swim every day. I walk. I'm also a vegetarian, and I don't drink. While I don't want people to give up the joys of youth, I do think you ought to prepare a bit for getting old. Just like you should save for being old, save your health as well. Enjoy yourself, but don't destroy your body.

*Have you always been careful of your health?*

Not as careful as I should have been, but I've always exercised and always eaten fairly sensibly. I suppose for the last five years I've been a vegetarian.

*Have you felt your memory getting worse?*

Yes, I do get forgetful. But I always say to people—since, of course, Bill died of Alzheimer's—not to get overly worried about it. This also is a natural phenomenon. I even say that to the kids, which they find valuable. Just pause, don't worry about it, and it'll pop back.

I never had a wonderful memory—Bill had a marvellous memory—it's not as good as it was, but it's still not that bad. So I get by. I do think that it was Bill's death that did this to me. It undermined my confidence a lot, and older people do lose their confidence. That's a worry. It's very important that you don't lose your self-respect; but, because we live in a young world, it does tend to happen to old people.

*Do you think that a lot of this we do to ourselves? We accept the stereotypes; we buy into them?*

Oh yes, I think so. But it is changing. I go swimming and walking at Bondi, and I'm seventy-four, and I think some of the people I see down there exercising would be ten years older than me. I almost feel like going and giving them a pat and a kiss because I'm so pleased. I do think that there is a different image of older people like, say, my grandma, who wore long black clothing. But I go out in shorts, I get around without shoes.

That brings me to another point that I feel is good about age. You don't care what people think [laughter], and that's very valuable. I see it down at the beach, and I certainly see it in myself. I just do not care. It isn't that I am rude to people; in fact, I think I'm more tolerant. I wear what I want to and, while I've never been a fashion plate—far from it—nowadays I feel I've got to be comfortable and do what I want. That applies to other things, I'm not going out to things—although I'm still in quite a number of organisations—or doing things I don't want to do. From time to time, things will come up in organisations I am in, and people (particularly younger people) pressure you. Somebody said quite recently, 'Don't make excuses and don't explain.' [laughter] And I say that to myself. By the time you reach seventy-four, you have got the right to do that.

*Do you find yourself being more selective about what you do, because you have less time?*

I cut my cloth according to how much energy I have. I know that by the evening I am not so energetic any more, whereas once upon a time I was out at meetings all night. Five years ago, I was still president of the Women's International Democratic Federation: I was travelling all over the world; I was going to meetings; I was presenting our point of view overseas and at two or three United Nations' special conferences on peace. I don't know whether it was Bill's death that did it, or whether seventy-four is a big change, but I couldn't sit up at night writing and preparing speeches.

*Are you still a member of the Communist Party?*

I don't think there is a Communist Party any more, Anne! But I am still a communist. However, I am re-thinking whether the communist doctrine included too much emphasis on development, and whether or not you've got to look at its impact on the environment and our lifestyles. Do we need development to give us as much as we've got? Shouldn't we start changing our expectations? It's ridiculous what so many of us have in the West while people have nothing in other countries. With the advance of communications, people will get to know that, and I think it's going to create problems. We have to be willing to share more. The fact that some people accumulate tremendous wealth is immoral. When you get to my age, you wonder what you want to accumulate it for. It's crazy, and I believe that society has to change. I still basically believe in Marxist philosophy. I think Marx and Engels were very profound thinkers, and people criticise superficially without reading what they wrote.

*What do you feel now about the way Australia is moving? Optimistic?*

I think we should be giving more attention to the poorer countries of the world and the poorer people in our own country. There is still too much concentration of wealth in too few hands; that's what worries me. I'm quite happy about us turning towards Asia, but I am not happy about us having military pacts with Indonesia, where there is such a denial of human rights. And all the aid money we pour into Papua New Guinea—a lot of it goes to the military to suppress the struggles of the people.

In comparison to other countries, much is done here for the benefit of people; but not enough goes into education. Our public education system is deteriorating. I am worried about the health system, and I am worried about superannuation. Is it being wisely invested? When the time comes, when people should be getting superannuation or the pension, will it have been squandered?

*You clearly keep very much abreast of everything that is going on. Do you read a lot?*

Yes, I do very much so, and that's one of the problems of getting old. I've always had excellent eyesight; I could read the tiniest print. I didn't see so well in the distance, but good enough. But now I've got to go to the doctor tomorrow because I can't read the very small print any more. I resent that. Seventy-four years I have done without glasses. I hate to think that I may have to have an operation or have glasses.

Mostly I watch the news, listen to the ABC, watch Channel Two and, of course, read.

*Do you think about what might happen in the next ten years?*

Personally, no, but I suppose it's in my mind. Some people buy into retirement villages, but I'm of the opinion we should stay in the community. I hope I never have to go into a nursing home. I only hope I drop dead. Now I live my life from day to day. I don't plan very far ahead. I get pleasure from my daughter and my grandchildren, and out of simple things like swimming and walking. And I still work in some organisations.

*Is there anything about death and dying that you fear?*

Like all people, I don't want to suffer. I would like to remain independent. My dad went just like that—dropped dead. With mum, it was a longer period. Bill had Alzheimer's. My brother died of cancer; he suffered in hospital for about two months. That was awful. I hated that because he was such an independent man. I hope that doesn't happen to me, but I don't think about it. I try to keep healthy, I have a check on all the things you should check on. As far as death is concerned, wasn't it Shakespeare who said, 'The poor beetle we tread on in mortal suffering feels the same pain as when a giant dies.' Death itself is nothing! It's just changing over from one state to another. It's the suffering before death that I hope I don't have to go through, or the loss of my independence.

*Do you feel that there is any part of you that will survive after your death, or do you believe that when you are dead, you are dead?*

I think that when you are dead, you are dead, and that's it. The only part of me that survives is some little spark that I've passed on to Lee and the grandkids I guess. So to that extent I suppose there is a little bit there. I think you come into being and you go out of being. When Bill died, he was cremated. Then, because he loved Bondi, we took his ashes there, and sprinkled them around the rocks. I look there every day.

*Can you talk about the beginning of the illness and what happened?*

It's one of the most frightful things that can happen to you. It's not only old people, because others get it when they're in their forties. Bill quite extraordinarily diagnosed himself. He was always forgetful—like, if I said on the way home, 'Bill, buy this,' he'd get home and say that he'd been too busy. But he never forgot an appointment. He didn't forget telephone numbers. He kept his mind in the direction he wanted it. So he must have noticed it, and he said to me, 'I wonder if I've got Alzheimer's?' I argued with him for two months that he had always been forgetful, till I then started to notice it. But other people noticed it as long as a year or eighteen months before. He was at meetings, and he would forget what he was saying. It's a dreadful complaint. To begin with, it doesn't seem to be hardly anything. And then when you read about what can happen, I could hardly believe that the time would come when Bill would be incontinent, that he'd lose control of his bowels, and that he wouldn't be able to walk or wouldn't be able to feed himself. And then gradually, of course, this does happen.

One of the very important things that I would campaign for is an extension of day care for people with disabilities. Bill was in a day-care program. He was picked up by bus of a morning, and he used to be away from 9.00 am till 2.30 pm. So I had a break and he had stimulation, because you can't give them that when you are exhausted. For the last six months of his life there were many nights when I had no sleep. I am still not over that.

*Is this because he didn't sleep?*
You would never know what was going to happen. It's heartbreaking. He would come in, switch my light on, and say, 'Oh, I've been looking for you everywhere and I couldn't find you. Where have you been?' You were always worried about what was going to happen—not that he ever wandered, but a few times he tried to open the front door. He did have accidents: he fell over and split his head open, and broke his shoulder, and things like that. But then, when something had happened, I'd get him back into bed and he'd go off to sleep. But I could never go back to sleep because I was so churned up.

*Was he frightened of what was going to happen when he found out he had the illness?*
Yes, I think he was very frightened. Of course, he went down to the library and read everything. He knew everything about it, and from what he read he thought it would be about ten years. It was much quicker than that. Instead of having it for four years, he probably had

it for about six. I remember when he did an interview for the film that was made about Alzheimer's, he sat down in front of the typewriter and said, 'You see, I can still type, but nonsense just comes out.'

*So he knew it was nonsense?*

Well, in the reasonably early stages he was still writing articles. He wrote this article and brought it to me. And I thought to myself, how am I going to handle this? He said, 'Well, what do you think? It's nonsense, isn't it?' I said, 'Yes, love, it's nonsense.' He said, 'That happens now. Everything I write is just nonsense.' I'm convinced he knew everything that was happening to him. You could almost see it in the eyes of people who have got Alzheimer's; they know something terrible is happening to them.

*I remember my mother, when I went back to England and she had already been diagnosed, saying, 'I'm in a fog, and you have come to rescue me.' So you do go through those awful emotional maelstroms, don't you? How did you support yourself?*

When he was diagnosed, I thought, my God! I don't know how I am going to handle this. So I read all I could about it. I took up yoga, and that helped me tremendously. When he went to day care, I would go and do yoga. As I walked up the steps I'd tell myself, 'Just relax.' And usually I did. I think that saw me through, because it's very hard physically, mentally, and emotionally caring for someone. For people who care, you can't pay enough tribute to them. It really is very, very difficult. What has me very worried today is that they are cutting back on home and community services. The authorities say, 'Keep people at home.' That's right, but society needs to provide more assistance. And the fact is, when you're minding a person—I'm speaking about Alzheimer's, although it applies to other carers as well—you are on duty twenty-four hours a day; more, it seems. You have to be able to have a break, or you will have a break-down.

*What did you find about community attitudes towards Alzheimer's?*

It differs. I had a very bad experience in this street where a woman rang up because of a disagreement—and I've always got on well with all my neighbours—and said Bill ought to be put away, it was bad for the street, and it was lowering the value of the houses. Which was utterly ridiculous, because no one would have known Bill even had

Alzheimer's. But even if there was a problem, it's terrible that someone would say such a thing. At first I said, 'Let me explain.' And then she said something, so I just slammed the phone down and tried to put it out of my mind. But obviously, I haven't put it out of my mind because I think it was such an awful thing to say. In general, we were always very open about it. Bill always said, 'I've got Alzheimer's', and I always said if I was anywhere, 'My husband has Alzheimer's.'

*What was the hardest thing for you in living with Bill through his illness?*
Seeing him lose his independence. It got to the stage where I was doing everything: I was bathing him, I had to wipe him after he went to the toilet, clean his teeth, wash him, and everything. That was terrible for all of us. Everyone likes to be independent, and he was such an independent man. Seeing him lose his capacity to express himself—because he was very articulate—his capacity to write, to see all that being lost, you know. When dad died, he just woke up one morning and said to mum, 'What's the time?' and he was gone. I would give ten years of my life to die like that instead of dying like Bill, or Leon, my brother who died of cancer.

*From the way you talk, you so clearly had a strong and close marriage over fifty years. Why do you think it worked for you when for so many people marriage is not working?*
I think you learn to give and take. I am very hot-tempered; Bill was very tolerant. But also, frankly, having the same political outlook helped us tremendously, because we always had so much to share. I can remember we would walk up and down Bondi Beach, and we'd 'solve' all the problems of the world. Life was never a bore.

*What did you learn from Bill during your lifetime with him?*
He taught me to drive a car. That was a very difficult period because I can remember Lee, my daughter, sitting in the back saying, 'I've never heard you fighting so much,' because he would get impatient with me and then I'd get cranky. He did teach me a lot to do with writing. Most important of all, he taught me the need for a tolerant attitude. He always saw the positive in people. He used to say, 'I'm too easy-going, and then suddenly people do something and I find I've got to stand up and have a fight about it.' So his tolerance and his easy-going

attitude to life had an impact on me. And I might say his extraordinary discipline. When he was writing—he wrote a number of books—he would get up at three in the morning and write, because he said that was the time when nothing disturbed him. My daughter has learned those qualities from him. She is also extremely disciplined.

*Did you learn anything from his illness?*

Yes, although there was a great deal of pain and suffering, I learned patience and tolerance, I learned to adapt, to try and find a way to explain. Because people with Alzheimer's do become tense and anxious, and I learned not to get into arguments. I can remember once we went through this terrible period, because I tried not to interfere so as to keep him as independent as long as possible. But sometimes he would put his pyjama trousers on his arms and three shirts, and I'd say, 'Bill, come on darling, take that off.' 'Right. If you say that, I'll do it. But what you've got to remember is, yours isn't the only point of view!' And so I'd try and explain. I say to those who are looking after people with Alzheimer's, 'Arguments arise, but you have to walk away from them. You cannot win. It's utterly illogical, so you have to find another way.' And that's very difficult.

*Did it affect the way you think about the value of human life?*

I think I have always valued human life. As I say, when I was very young the idea of war, or that people were hungry and suffering, really stirred me up. But I suppose Bill's suffering reinforced the idea that the most important thing to have is your health and independence. You can have all the money, all the possessions in the world; but if you lose that independence and become utterly reliant on someone else, it's a terrible thing. That is why now I almost excessively want to be independent, because I've seen the pain and anguish that dependency brings to people.

*Is there such a thing as the essence of a person that remains, do you think? Even with an illness like Alzheimer's?*

From what I have read and heard, some people change completely. I can only speak of Bill, and he didn't. As you put it, the essence was there, until a few days before he died when Lee and I were trying to get him to walk—because we tried to keep him moving. When we were talking he still would say, 'What are you doing about it?' His desire to organise things, to see that something was done wherever there was injustice—that was still there. The last few months of his life he was in a nursing home, and he was really fantastic. That concern for other people was still there, although you had to try to clean his teeth, and feed him, etc. But he was so concerned about keeping himself tidy, even when he was so ill, and his face would light up when Lee and his grandchildren walked in.

*The other thing you were talking about was the way he would go to the day-care centre and come back with all their papers, because papers had obviously been so much a part of his life.*

Yes. I think a lot of people who have Alzheimer's do maintain what they've done all their life. Bill was always a writer and he loved it, so he would go to the day centre and collect their documents. They used to say, 'We try to check, but when he comes home would you also check him?' And often we'd find that he had brought home their papers. God only knows how, and even then he would sit down and go through them as if he was correcting them. He was still trying to write, a year or eighteen months after he was diagnosed.

*With my mother's Alzheimer's, she had been a designer, so visual things were very important, and that stayed with her. She had also been a very sociable woman, and that stayed with her—sometimes with unexpected consequences. I remember once when three dozen cases of sherry arrived, followed by half the local shopkeepers whom she'd invited in for drinks. Another time, she came down to a party my brother was giving for his new boss, and she had dressed up for the occasion in a black jumper, black bloomers, black stockings, a huge Parisian hat covered with roses, and wearing all her jewellery, brooches, necklaces, earrings, and rings on every finger. Everybody acted as if it was all perfectly normal.*

Oh, isn't that lovely! I was telling Anne, Lee, about dad and his pyjama trousers ... [Freda's daughter, Lee, had joined us at this point.]

Lee: Did you tell her about the time at the Opera House?

Oh, no, I forgot to tell her that. We went down to the Opera House, and he said, 'I want to go to the toilet.' I said, 'Okay,' so he went to the toilet at the Opera House and came out with his trousers folded over his arm. I said, 'Bill, what on earth are you doing?' He said, 'You told me to take them off.' And I said, 'Darling, go back in the toilet and put them on.' And he said once again, 'If you say so, but I don't know why one minute you say take them off and the next minute you say put them back on.' [laughter] Everybody looked in the other direction.

*Do you think there is a changed attitude?*

Yes. Things are more open. There is more acceptance. However, I do think the government has made a mistake, in that everyone is out in the community. I don't think they're prepared for it. Some of them are not well-cared for, and they are suffering.

*Are you working now?*

Yes. I want to tell you about something we are doing here in the senior media network. It will be interesting to see how it goes. We go to schools and talk to the students. We suggest to the kids that they bring some photos of their grandparents or old friends—photos of when they were children, when they were adolescent, when they were working, or in the army or what you will, and now they are old. Then we will talk to the children about what it is like being old, and ask them to draw an old person, which the council has agreed to display.

**Dorothy Buckland-Fuller, who came from a Greek family, was talking about old people not being separated from their communities, and children being encouraged to touch old skin, which often doesn't happen here.**

I think that's very important. My daughter has encouraged her three kids to kiss me and hug me, because otherwise people are often afraid of an old person, which is very sad. I think they even feel at my age I'm a bit of a comfort. I was bringing my grandson home—I used to collect him when he was in infants—and one day Lee came home from Uni and she was looking for me, and the lady next door said, 'She is up the street sailing boats in the gutter with a little boy.' Thinking back, when I used to pick Lee up from kindy, I was always in a hurry to get home, buy something, and make tea. But with Conor and the grandkids, I've got time, and they know I have time.

**Do people ever talk down to you because they think you are old and not of any consequence?**

I'm glad you asked that, because some people, they really don't know how to talk to an older person. Some people are almost afraid. They shy away from you. I don't know necessarily whether it is widespread, but sometimes I have felt offended because I feel they really have patronised me.

*Is this just people you meet socially, or does it happen through work?*
Well, I mentioned this Alzheimer's committee I am on, which has mostly professionals—doctors, social workers, etc—and at times I have felt that they are patronising. I was there to represent the elderly, but I never felt I was part of it. So I resigned. I had experience that was valuable, and I should have stayed and found the way to express it!

*I know you said that you didn't plan ahead. But how would you like to live in this next phase of your life?*
I am still concerned about people, and about society. When you have been like that all your life it doesn't go away. I hope to continue the work that I am doing in health for older people, and for older people to be represented in a better way in the media. I am not only doing it for myself. When my daughter and my grandchildren get old, I want them to have a dignity and respect that I haven't had—that's not quite correct—that some old people don't have. I want old people to have their position in society. So I hope to work on committees like that and, bang, just suddenly to drop dead! And not to have a long illness and to be dependent and a pest.

*How would you like to be remembered?*
It doesn't matter much. You've lived your life; you have passed on. I've not made any enormous contribution to society. For a while, I hope Lee and my grandchildren will think about me with affection. But that doesn't matter, either. You come and go.

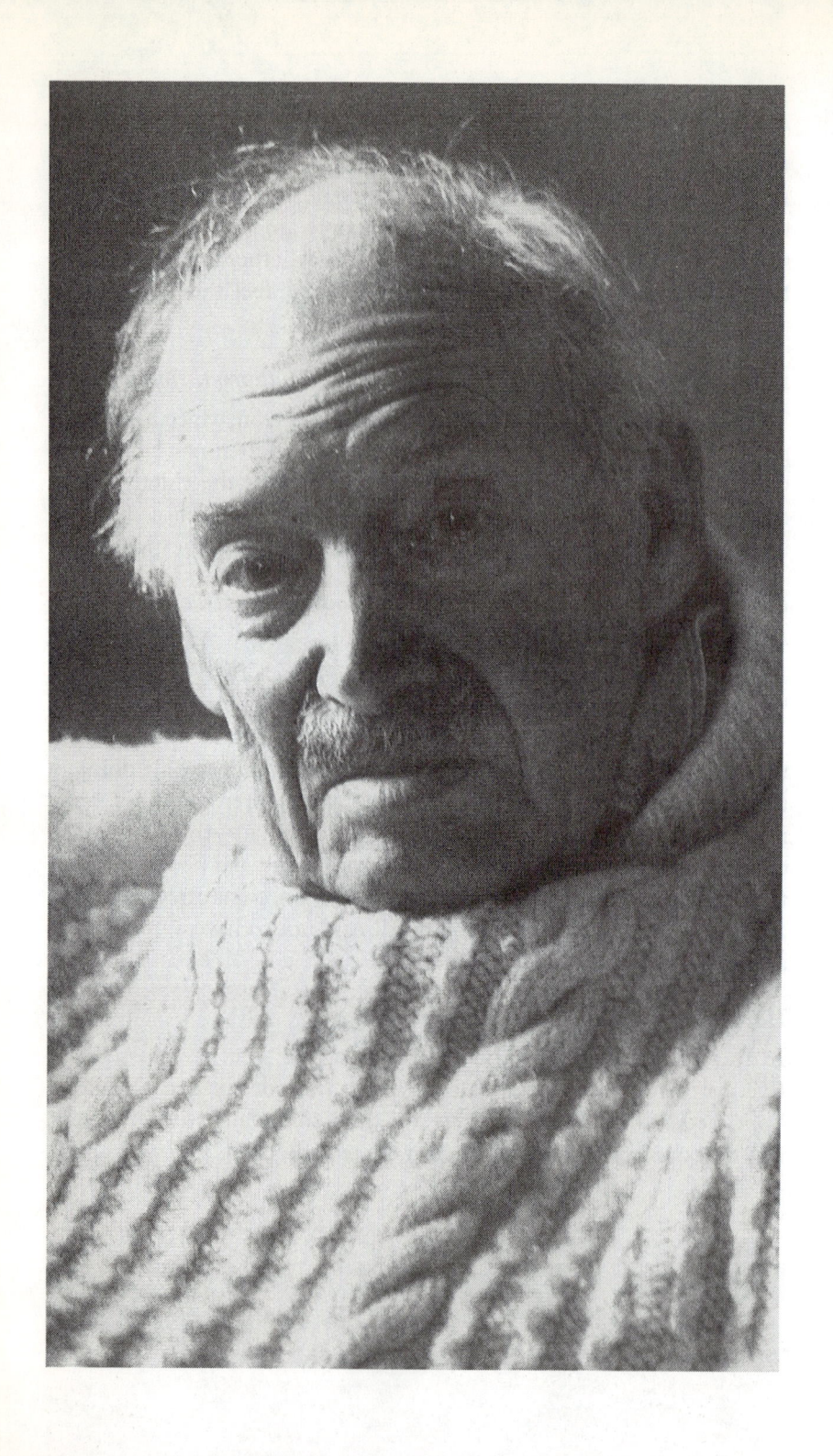

# John Bray
*I don't recommend it*

John Jefferson Bray AC, QC was born in Adelaide in 1912, and is one of South Australia's most distinguished citizens—a lawyer, scholar, writer, and poet. He was educated at the Sevenhill Primary School, St. Peter's College, and the University of Adelaide from where he graduated with a Bachelor of Law degree, later becoming a Doctor of Law. He was Chief Justice of South Australia from 1967 to 1978, and Chancellor of the University of Adelaide from 1968 to 1983. He was made a Companion of the Order of Australia in 1979.

John Bray has published five collections of poetry and two collections of poetry, prose, and public addresses. *Satura* (poetry and prose) won the South Australia Festival Award for Literature in 1990. His last volume of poetry, *Seventy Seven*, was published in 1990, and includes recent poems, European translations, and adaptations from the Greek. It is dedicated to his colleagues, the Friendly Street Poets, 'For comradeship, example and survival.' Several of Bray's later poems relate to the reality of human finitude, and he observes his own ageing with a wry candour. He lives in an old bluestone terrace house within the city precincts of Adelaide.

I had elderly relations when I was a child, but I never thought I'd be one of their number eventually. Both my parents lived to be over eighty, and so did my grandmother. Of course, I remember them.

*Were you conscious of your parents becoming old?*

Not until I was middle-aged myself, when they started to fail; until then I just regarded them as people. They were obviously getting older, but it didn't impinge on me.

*What do you remember of your father?*

Oh ... it's hard to say. I lived with him until he died, and I lived with my mother until she died after that. We had a ... I don't know, a modus vivendi, I suppose you would call it. I was never very close to him.

*Was your father a lawyer?*

No, he was all sorts of things. He was a sharebroker for many, many years, and then he had a fruit block at Penwortham. I lived up there as a child for some years; then he retired, quite early.

*You talked about a period in your middle age when you became conscious of getting older. How did that happen?*

Oh, when I was forty I thought I was getting into old age; when I was fifty I was certain I was at least middle aged. But I seemed to get younger when I retired. In many ways they were the best years of my life, from my late sixties, early seventies—I was free from responsibility, free from having to work, doing anything I didn't want to do, and I still felt vigorous, healthy, young. I used to swim a lot, walk a lot. Can't do those things now.

*Did you worry about getting older?*

In the last four or five years I started to think about it more and more as my activities were necessarily reduced. It's a great nuisance not being able to walk as I used to. I get out of breath—I've got emphysema. Ordinary household tasks seem to take longer and be more tedious [pauses]. I still walk up to Hutt Street; I'm going up there after this interview to do the week's shopping. How long it will last I don't know.

*Are there advantages in getting older?*

I don't think so. I don't recommend it. There is an optimum point, I think, when you're free of the necessity of earning a living and you still feel young and vigorous. I still think it was a good time.

*So, it's the physical frailties that are the irksome ones?*
Well, I imagine mental ones would be much worse. But I flatter myself, perhaps foolishly, that I haven't suffered any mental degeneration, though I notice that I forget things more than I used to. Fortunately, they are not important. I forget where I've put things. I forget people's names, sometimes, even when I remember their faces. But still, these are quite common sort of things.

*Does it make you anxious?*
No. If it got seriously worse it would make me anxious; but at the moment it's only a minor irritation. As for forgetting people's names, they're mostly people's names I don't want to remember, anyhow.

*One of the advantages it seems to me, as you get older, is that you cease to mind as much about what people think about you, or about what you do.*
I've never cared much; and I don't care about it at all now, subject to the law.

*I recall my father, who never cared much either, but who certainly was a very withdrawn man. When he was about seventy he developed lung cancer, and became the kind of person who you always felt was there inside; he became a man of great wit and exuberance, and it was almost as if his whole personality blossomed because he didn't care any longer.*
That's right. That is one of the advantages of getting older. You simply don't care, and you don't care if people see that you don't care.

*What about friendships? Do you feel they are as important as they were?*
Yes. Fortunately, I've always been able to make friends with people younger than myself—besides, of course, my contemporaries and people older than myself.

*Were you a vain man?*

I don't think I was vain about my physical appearance. I was vain about academic robes and things like that.

*Thinking about age today, there appears to be a cult of youth, particularly in television.*

I don't watch the media. At least, I haven't got a television set [pauses]. Sometimes I envy youth. I envy the vigour and the good looks.

*Again, it wasn't very long ago when most people didn't live to three score years and ten; it's possible that those who did survive were more venerated. Now, old people are often regarded as a problem.*

I suppose they are. I hope I'm not a problem, but if I am I'm not conscious of it and I don't care. I'm not a burden on anyone. At least I don't think I am, financially anyhow.

*Did you plan for getting older?*

I can't say that I did consciously, no. When I came to this house twenty odd years ago, I decided to sleep downstairs, which I've always done. Ah... even then I found the stairs a bit irksome. I thought, why should I go up and down them more than I have to? So I do all my living downstairs. You've got to realise that the disappearance of the domestic servant, which happened in my lifetime, has made a great difference to one's lifestyle. Advantages and disadvantages. You don't have to keep up appearances before the servants, because there aren't any servants to keep up appearances before. Well, I do find things like washing up more irksome than I used to, but that's only because it's boring and repetitive.

*Do you ever use being old to your advantage?*

Yes. I'm able to refuse a lot of things now that I would have felt morally bound to accept in years gone by. In fact, I had pleasure in writing a letter this week refusing an invitation to a formal dinner, saying I have reached the age—over eighty—where I can't attend such functions with any satisfaction to myself or pleasure to anyone else.

*Do you seek solitude more now?*

Yes, I do.

*It is supposed to be a characteristic of getting older that people think*

*more and more about their past. Has that happened to you?*
I've always been intensely historically minded and interested in civilisations of the past. Still am. But if you mean living in my own past, I don't know that I do very much. I think about past events, of course. I suppose everyone does.

*Are there events or periods that stand out for you?*
Well I am a student of the classics, particularly interested in Greek and Roman literature. I've written a lot of adaptations of Greek poems. I'm interested in all the books that are coming out now about the figures of the last hundred years or so of the nineteenth century, the Victorian era in particular.

*What gave you your interest in history? Has it been with you from childhood?*
Yes. Partly it's the colour and flamboyance.

*But not all history presumably is colourful or flamboyant?*
Oh no, no. I'm not interested in economic history. My grandmother lived in the nineteenth century, and had a staff of servants and regulated hours. I stayed with her from time to time when my parents went to England, when I was an adolescent, and on various other occasions, and I got the feel of Victorian life.

*Would you like to have lived in that period?*
No. The restraints of convention were much greater then. I don't think I could have borne having to dress for dinner every night, and 'Not before the servants'. But my grandmother was used to that. She used to say with an air of modest pride, 'I can't even make a cup of tea'. Nor could she.

*Do people treat you differently because you are old?*
Yes, in a way. They give me seats. Help me up the stairs and that sort of thing. Of course, I'm no longer treated with respect as a judge. That's rather pleasing.

*But people don't treat you as if you're losing your marbles? I wouldn't think they would dare.*
Sometimes, when I go into a reverie, people say, 'Are you still there,

are you listening, are you with us?' I say, 'Yes, yes, yes, go on.'

*So when you do go into those reveries, are they usually do to with your work?*
No. I'm just letting my mind wander with free association and various things. But I can abstract myself from a conversation if I'm not interested in it.

*Have you always been able to do that?*
Oh, yes. Always, or quite often, if I've been with people who are interested in races or football or cricket—which I am not, I just switch off.

*You talk about history. What have you learned from history?*
Oh, I suppose if I must pick out one factor, I'd say that it was realisation of how unchanging human nature is, despite the various forms and fashions of particular periods.

*Do you think that you have changed, or are you conscious of an essential John Bray that's remained there since childhood?*
I haven't thought of that, but I've changed with the greater freedom of social attitudes. I have changed enormously. I remember when I was first made Chief Justice, there was a picture of me in the paper going down to the beach on Sunday in casual gear, which many people thought indecorous at the time. Nobody would think anything of it now.

*Yes, you've also talked about the irksomeness of constraints. Is this something that's concerned you all your life?*
Yes, but the restraints have got less and less.

*Do you think about death much?*
It's in the back of my mind. I can't say I brood over it all the time.

*How do you regard it?*
Oh, I'm a sceptic. It's possible, of course, there's an afterlife. But I think the odds are against it.

*Do you have or have you had any particular faith?*

Not since I grew up, no.

*Did you have a religious upbringing?*

No, but I was confirmed and prepared for confirmation. That prayer that says, 'I always promise that when two or three are gathered together in my name I will grant what they ask'—something like that, anyhow. I read that and I thought, I'll try this out in church one day. There were certainly more than one or two or three gathered together in the name of God, and I expressed my wishes and they didn't come true. And I thought: well, perhaps one shouldn't take these things literally. Anyhow, don't put your trust in it.

*Don't put your trust in God, but trust in yourself? Have you had trust in yourself?*

For ordinary life, yes. I haven't trusted myself always to behave prudently and discreetly and soberly or righteously.

*How do you remember yourself as a small boy?*

Oh, I played, I read a lot. I didn't like school, I didn't like compulsory sport, which I thought was ridiculous and still think ridiculous. I was not very gregarious as a child, because I didn't share the interests of my contemporaries. I've been much more gregarious since I grew up.

*And as a man in the prime of your life? What recollections do you have then?*

That's hard to say. Of course, I was very busy and worked very hard in my profession. Being a QC absorbed a large proportion of my energies. But I did what most men do: I played a bit, drank a lot, read a lot.

*And now, is there work that you still want to do?*

Oh yes, I'd like to see my latest book, a life of the Roman Emperor, Gallienus, into the press, and I still write poetry.

*Has the nature of your poetry changed?*

Yes I think it has. Certainly the theme of death does seem to be prominent there. Perhaps I exorcise that by writing about it.

*How would you like to be remembered?*

Oh as a writer, a good companion, I hope a good judge, I'm not sure about that. How would I know? [pauses] I trust that my intimate friends will all remember me with affection. No doubt the memory will dim with time. Perhaps my works will live after me, I hope so. But who knows? Fashions in literature change.

***Which of your poems would you like to read?***

'Consolation to Remus.' As you know, Romulus and Remus were brothers. They founded Rome. Romulus built the wall. Remus in mockery jumped over it, and Romulus killed him.

### Consolation to Remus

> It was wrong, of course, to jump and jeer at your brother's wall.
> For a wall is a sacred barrier, only with ritual crossed,
> And he who despises and spurns it spurns the gods of the state and the hearth.
> So he struck you down, and rightly, your common conception forgotten,
> And the thin sharp milk of the she-wolf, and the reek of her fur in the rain,
> And the perils shared and the prizes, and the wicked uncle dispatched
> So you have no part in the glory, in the high imperial column,
> The seemly chorus of children, the trumpet, the wreath and the triumph,
> The senators togaed in purple, the pontifex placid and holy,
> The roads that run like spokes from the Capitolian hub
> To the rock-bound rim of the world as it rolls with the rule of law.
> These for the children of Romulus: trellised vines on the risen wall.
>
> For walls make civil compartments: they classify heaven and earth,
> Grading off right and rank, the regions of men and the gods,
> The native-born and the stranger, the pilots and cargo of power,
> Passable only at checkpoints, subject to stamp and toll
> The transit tallied and sanctioned by the guardians, grave at the gate.
> Yet you have your role in the story, your half of the seed of the god,
> Identical twin with Romulus, haired tail to his stately head.
> His the open and civic, the ceremonial cloak,
> Yours the hooded and hidden, the sweat and the stain on the shirt,
> The grin and the spit in the gutter, the jerk of the upturned thumb.
> For walls are reared to be leapt and barriers built to be burst,
> And Clodia creeps from the bed of the consul and swerves
> from the verse of Catullus,
> And pads to the peeling streaming tetterous tenement wall,

And there, in the dark, in the alley, obliges your gap-toothed sons.
There are you justified, Remus: there is your mural crown.

***I like that. Why did you pick that one?***
I don't know. I like it, too. Here's another:

### The Persimmons

Six tawny globes crowned with black polar stars,
Burn on the bowl: their taut translucent skin
Rather promotes than veils what lies within,
Like Vulcan's net when Venus tangled Mars.
Now prove these promised joys. Taste one and try.
What scraping bitterness, what clawed acridity,
What griping, green, unseasoned, thin acidity,
The palate ploughed, the puckered lip awry.
But wait: wait till the crackled stars turn brown,
The slackened skins in sagging scrollwork creep,
Or stickily in oozy patches weep.
Then boldly bite. The luscious flesh glides down.
So those to whom fair-seeming youth proves sour
In shrivelled age may see their sweetness flower.

***Last time, we were talking about history, and your awareness that human nature hasn't changed. Do you think we are better in any way, though?***
Yes, in some ways. I think we treat animals better, and there's less racism, less anti-feminism. But on the other hand there are all these horrific crimes that keep on getting committed. Perhaps, you know, we lose here and gain there.

***Yes. It's interesting if you look at legislation and social mores, there are some behaviours that we now say are not acceptable any longer.***
But on the other hand—

***Look what we do in wars everywhere?***
—Yes. But then we have much more sexual freedom. Abortion is legal. Homosexuality is legal. Whether these things are improvements or not, of course, is a matter of opinion. I think some of them are and some aren't. I'd like to read:

### Invocation

Terminus, God of the boundaries, keeper of fence and line,
See to my life's compartments, lest their colours cross and combine,
Or the springs and wells of the passions be choked with professional dust,
Or the laurels and vines of the Muses be strangled by tendrils of lust.
Janus, God of beginnings, and so of endings too,
Looking forwards and backwards, holding future and past in review,
Sever my chapters cleanly, clear one's feet from his foregoer's skirt,
Grant penultimate Indian summer, and let the last scene be curt.

Lords of the mete-wand and hour-glass, dealers in fortunes and lucks,
Stamping illusions of patterns on the queasy cosmic flux,
Time is an endless ladder, space is an endless plain,
Carve me a gracious portion, cut it along my grain.

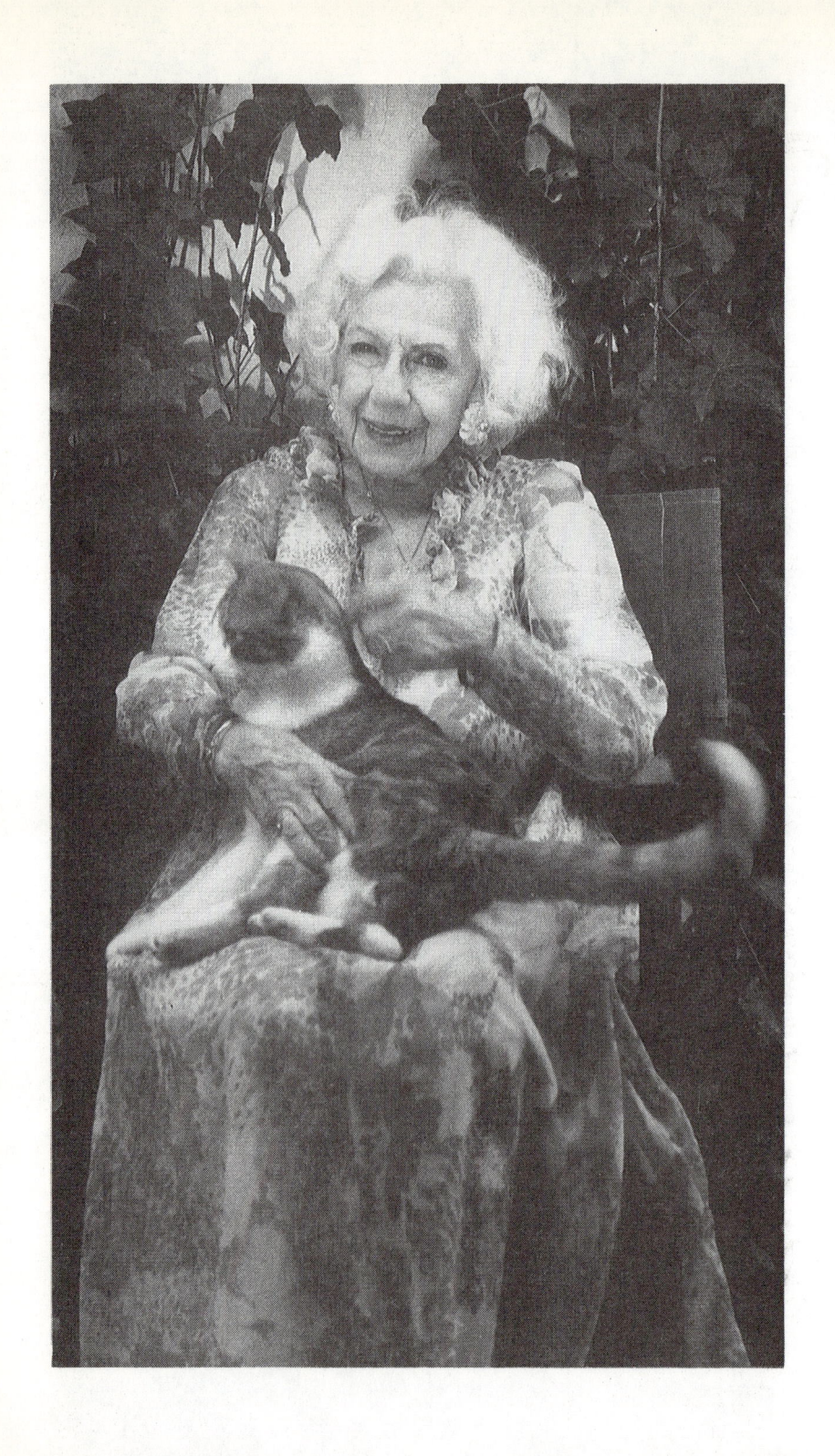

# Colleen Clifford
*I'm so lucky*

Colleen Clifford, well into her nineties, and grande dame of Australian theatre, has enjoyed over seventy years working in musicals, drama, variety, cabaret, television, and radio. Her film credits include *Careful, He Might Hear You*, *The Coca Cola Kid*, and *The Year My Voice Broke*. Her one-woman show, *A Nightingale Still At It In Berkeley Square*, was performed at the Sydney Opera House in 1992 to standing ovations. In 1994 she received another standing ovation when she was given the highest of the coveted 'Mo' Awards.

Clifford was born in England, in November 1898, the same year that Pierre and Marie Curie announced the discovery of radium and polonium, Count Ferdinand von Zeppelin built the world's first airship, the Paris Metro was opened, and the first photographs were taken utilising artificial light.

Colleen Clifford now lives in Australia. When I met her, she had spent the night before taking two friends to the theatre, followed by supper, and had then read through the night until ten past five in the morning. She said she was not at all tired. She lives at the back of a small terrace house in Paddington which she shares with two actor friends, an unruly puppy, and two cats. Her room could only belong to someone who has spent her life in the theatre. I have an impression of rows of dresses, sequins and tulle, hats and hat boxes, make-up in all its bottles and tubes and vials, and hundreds of photographs. She is still performing and teaching.

God gave me vitality, and I'm doing what I've always done. Just because I'm in my nineties, it's not dawned on me to sit and say, 'I am getting old, and now I must stop.' It's only my knees, which I did in through a riding accident years ago, that sometimes bother me. Before that, I've danced and played tennis and high-kicked and ridden, but I think this last eighteen months arthritis must have set in, and now I look old as I walk, which isn't good for my vanity [laughs].

*But you don't feel any different inside?*
Not inside, no. You look at my diary. I go out to first nights, I've got engagements to sing, engagements to make films. So, you know, I'm very lucky.

*So you are still working professionally?*
Oh, yes. I'm doing one next Saturday and one the Sunday afterwards—that's my one-woman show—and for the last two years I've done my one-woman show at the Opera House. You see, I've worked all round Australia in a show I called, *A Nightingale Sings At Berkeley Square*. Then I did a second show and called it, *A Nightingale Still In Berkeley Square*. I thought, 'What the Dickens am I going to call the third one?' So I settled on, *A Nightingale Still At It In Berkeley Square*.

*What were you parents like? Did they have the same kind of vitality?*
They had a lot of vitality, and I adored them both. I had a father who was good-looking and danced like an angel, and a mother who had lots of vitality and was very fascinating. They were lovely to watch dancing together, ballroom dancing. They were full of fun. My father had a beautiful voice and sang, but nobody ever thought of my going on the stage. After all, you must remember I was born in 1898. So when I was growing up it wasn't the thing to be on the stage if you belonged to a good family.

*So your parents weren't on the stage?*
No, no, no. But from the age of three I danced and sang and carried on. My mother used to take me to all the music halls and the musical comedies. And then she thought she'd take me to a classical concert, so we went to the Albert Hall. After a quarter of an hour I said in clear ringing tones, 'Mummy, when's the funny man coming on?', which

shocked everyone. My father was in the army and, because his regiment went all over the place, my mother used to spend most of the time with him. Then she'd rush home, grab my brother and myself and a piano and a governess and a cook—they must have had money in those days—and whisk us off to the South of France or Brussels or somewhere. We had a lovely time. Sometimes she used to leave me with an aunt who was quite the reverse: very strict, but a wonderful old girl. Then my mother used to let me loose when she came back.

*Did your parents live to an old age?*
When the blitz was at its height we got them to some charming people who had a big farm in Shropshire, and my father died there at the age of seventy-six. Then, after twenty years of marriage, my husband, who I adored, died suddenly of a heart attack. We were still so much in love, I just couldn't bear England without him. My mother had come out here to visit my brother, and they both loved it so much that they had decided to stay. So I thought I'd join them for a couple of months, pull myself together, and return. When I was here, I discovered that my mother was suffering from osteoarthritis, and I was told that within two years she would be completely paralysed. I wasn't going to have her put in a nursing home, and I knew my brother and his wife wouldn't be able to look after her. So I thought, I don't care anything about a career. And I cancelled about a year's contracts in London, and stayed. I am pleased to say that she lived until she was three weeks short of ninety-three. She was completely paralysed by that time, but her eyes and her skin were good. I miss her terribly even still.

*How did you begin your career?*
When I was fifteen my father left the army because of ill health, and took us all out to New Zealand. I absolutely adored it, because the first thing he did was to buy a run, what we call a station here. I learned to muster sheep and drove cattle, and I thought I'd spend the rest of my life doing that. But in the meantime, during my early life I'd had great masters for the piano, and I was a pretty brilliant pianist. When the Royal Academy Examiners came to New Zealand, they gave me the gold medal for the highest mark in New Zealand, and then for the whole of Australasia. They also gave me a scholarship for the Royal Academy of Music. I had a lovely time at the Academy, but at the same time I was always getting things up for charity, and various directors

were offering me professional jobs. I decided for myself that it was a darn sight easier to sing and act on stage than spend six hours a day practising, much to the rage of the head of the Academy who said, 'We wasted two years on you if you're not going to be a concert pianist.' Anyhow, the piano has stood me in awfully good stead, because I became a variety artist among other things. I used to take the mickey out of pianists and operatic singers. I had an operatic soprano voice—coloratura—but now I'm a basso profundo!

*Do you look back over your life at all?*

Oh, I think I do. I've always got memories tottering into my head. I have a theory that I'm such a happy nature because we lived in a house that was full of love and fun and music, as well as full of discipline. I had two brothers. One was killed in the war—that's a picture of him when he was only eight—but I adored him. And my other brother is living in the Gold Coast.

*How old is he?*

He's eighty-nine. I am the oldest; I'm ninety-six. Two years ago, 'Column Eight' in the *Sydney Morning Herald* said I was ninety-five. I rang them up and said, 'How dare you take away the remaining drops of my youth. I'm ninety-four!'

*Going back to your childhood, which was such a happy one, what were your earliest memories?*

I can remember being held up by my mother at the age of three to talk to my father's brother officers at the mess. They used to say, 'Put your daughter up to sing,' and I used to sing, 'Hallo my baby, Hallo my honey, Hallo I'm all alone.' I can remember being taken to all the famous old comedians—Little Tich, Danleno, Florrie Ford, Vesta Tilley.

*Did you like clothes when you were a little girl?*

Yes. My mother used to dress me in the most beautiful party clothes. I remember going to one party, and coming down in a very pretty party frock, but then looking down at my feet I saw I still had on my galoshes over my little white kid shoes. I sat there petrified with humility and horror.

I can also remember, when we were very young, people being very shocked at my mother taking us all over the world to eat at different places. People were shocked; they said it was dreadful for children's digestions. 'Nonsense,' said my mother. 'It means that when they are grown up they can eat anything.' And that's true. I know grown-ups today who never touch this or never touch that. We ate curries, French food, Spanish food, any old thing.

*After your husband died, did you marry again?*
Never. We were so in love I couldn't dream of anybody else. It's a funny thing, but there is a great patch of being on stage in my life that is missing. When I married, I was already starring. But I decided that I would not go into any production, because I didn't want to go out of the house every night just as he came back. I never regretted it, because I had such a wonderfully happy married life. But because he loved music and theatre I was very lucky. I did cabaret and variety, and I'm a Royal Command performer, all that sort of thing. Then one day, about nineteen years after we'd been married, he heard me say on the phone, 'No, you know it's no use asking me to take part in a production,' and he said, 'Darling, I'm invalided out of the airforce now and I'm at home all day; I'd love you to go back on the stage.' So I said, 'Yes.' It was the big American production of *Guys and Dolls* with the whole American cast, and I was the third woman lead. I was in it right up to the night my husband died, and afterwards. And then I begged them to release me.

*Did you ever have children?*
No, I never had children. My husband was made air attaché to the British Embassy in Washington when Halifax was the ambassador. His assistant attaché was Roald Dahl—Stalky, we used to call him. Six foot three, and a character; a very brilliant mind, though. He came to see me in England and said, 'Air Commander has to have a hostess. You've got to come out.' So out I went, and we had two wonderfully interesting years. My husband managed to rent a house that he said was partly early Red Indian and partly early Elizabethan, but it had the most enormous sitting room. He bought me a grand piano, and we used to have the most gorgeous parties. When we left, my husband was given the highest award Americans can give a serving officer of another country.

*Have you ever been lonely?*

I suppose I've had my moments, but I can't remember them. You see, I'm an avid reader, and I am so glad to be alone so that I can read. God's been very good to me, he's enabled me to keep my spiritual faith. I happen to be a Catholic, and I believe so much in that lovely friend. We all have our moments of depression, but I say I know I'm all right; I'm with Him.

*And have you always had energy?*

I think I have. These confounded knees make me very tired when I'm walking now. You should see me get on a bus, oh God!

*Because your profession is one which has kept you much in the public eye, did you mind the change in your physical appearance as you grew older?*

Well, yes, but I don't think you're so aware of it until you look at an old picture. At the moment, everyone is laughing at me and saying I'm making such a fuss, because I'm horrid at the moment. I've got Panstick stuck all over black bruises, I've got a nose which has always been a fairly big one, but which makes me look like W C Fields, and now it's swollen and it's slightly crooked. I walked into the sitting room which has a hard parquet floor, tripped and fell from a standing position slap on to my nose. They X-rayed it and said it wasn't broken, but it was very painful.

*Do you think there is an essence of a person that stays the same, no matter what their age, whether they are nine or ninety?*

I think so. I don't think I've changed. I was always a bit bubbly, and I've kept the same love of things that are mystical, and love of reading and of music. I think that's why I haven't turned into [guying it] an ooold person [laughs].

*Did you ever think of having a face lift?*

Yes, I did. But then I thought, 'Oh what the hell!' It's a funny thing: there are days when you think, 'I don't look so bad,' and days when you think, 'Oh God!' You see, being on the stage, I have to think of my appearance. I have only aged very much in the last year. I was eight stone six, but I got like my old cat: I can only eat a very little at a time, whereas I used to have an enormous appetite. I've gone down to six stone one. It's extraordinary. There's a picture there of me when I was sixty, and you can see there is still quite a look of youth in the face.

*Are you conscious of only having limited time?*
I try not to think of it. It haunts me a little. It haunts me. Oh, somebody said something so sweet last night. They said, 'When you go to heaven, people will say, "What a long time you've been".' I thought that was lovely. They took it for granted I was going to heaven, mind you.

*Are there things you still want to do?*
I directed for the Edgeleys at His Majesty's in Perth. I directed six musical and two plays, and I'd love to direct one more. I had a great compliment paid me: I was asked when I was living in Perth to go to Melbourne to direct Noel Coward's latest musical. I had to refuse because I never left my mother at night. They bought Noel Coward out to direct it instead. Of course, I knew Noel Coward quite well. He was very witty but kind and charming. The only people he was unkind to were gushing people and very dull people. But he was so thoughtful; look, he left all his money to an orphanage for the children of stage people who had died. It was his idea and his great joy.

*Are there advantages to being old?*
Yes. People do half the work for you—oh yes, you can play on that [laughs].

*And disadvantages?*
Not being able to move quickly; not being able to walk quickly—but that's because of my blasted knees. I haven't found many other disadvantages. All my young people say, 'Oh, we never think of you as old, Miss Clifford.'

*Are you wiser?*
Oh, I hope I'm wiser. I would be a very stupid woman if I wasn't wiser.

*What have you learned that has been important to you?*
I've learned to be tolerant, to know that if someone seems to be absolutely beastly that there is a reason behind it. I've learned not to make snap judgements. Those are the sort of things I've learned.

*Is there any change in your enjoyment of life?*

I think I enjoy it just as much. You know, I get quite excited if something is happening. I look forward to going to parties.

*Some people I've talked to say they become a bit bored, a kind of ennui sets in because they think they've done it all before.*

This never sets in with me. For instance, at the moment I'm reading three books at the same time. I never have a dull moment, and of course I have my rosary to say. And I love my teaching—so many of the stars of the moment are trained by me.

*So are you a patient person?*

I am patient in teaching, but I don't think I am patient in ordinary life.

*What makes you angry?*

What makes me angry are people that are intolerant [roars of laughter].

*And what gives you the most pleasure?*

Lovely music, lovely acting, dear friends.

*Do you ever get frightened?*

No, I don't think so [pauses]. You ask such interesting questions. I suppose I have been frightened in my life, yes. New Zealand and the earthquakes used to frighten me, wobble wobble!

*I suppose I was thinking about whether you are frightened of being attacked, because you are little and you are old.*

I haven't thought about that. Someone has given me a wonderful gadget. It's standing there—you are attacked, and you press it, and it screams. It goes on for five minutes. But I've come to the conclusion that by the time I've opened my bag and found it, it would be too late.

*Are you frightened of dying?*

To be honest, I'm a split personality. My faith tells me that I shouldn't be. I don't want to die, and yet one part of me says, 'The eye has not seen nor ear heard.' I think one's nature says, 'Oh, I want to go on for ever.' But I don't think I'd like to become so decrepit. You see, my life's so full at the moment. It's very hard.

*Yes, I think a friend was saying you'd been up all night at a party, and yet you made an appointment to see her the next day at nine in the morning.*

Oh, I'm doing that all the time.

*Do people treat you differently now that you are older; are they ever condescending?*

Yes, in a way. But I'm quite pleased when I am given a chair and a cushion, and asked if I'm comfortable, all that sort of thing.

*How would you like to be remembered?*

This always surprises me. I have hundreds of letters and postcards (I never know where to put my hands on them, because I'm an untidy woman) saying that, through my happiness in life, I have helped so many people. That does make me happy. I sound awfully self-opinionated and vain, but God's been so good to me—lovely parents, adorable husband, good friends, and talent. I am lucky.

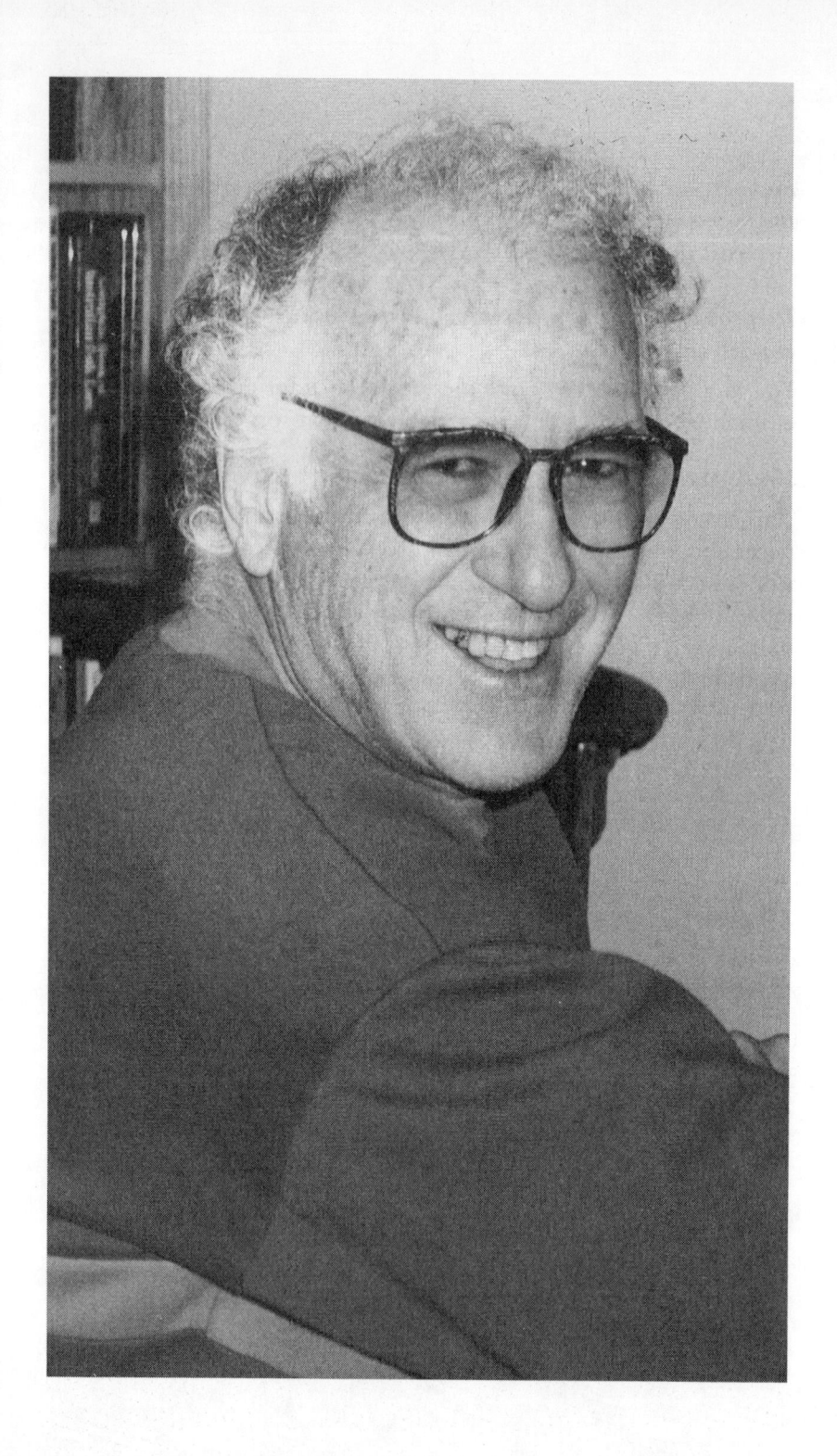

# Bernard Lake
*Making a choice*

Bernard Lake is a physician who for thirty years has specialised in helping people attain and maintain a high level of fitness. He was born in Sydney in May 1929, went to Sydney Boys' High and Sydney University, and studied and worked in London and Edinburgh before returning to Australia in 1957 and establishing himself as a consultant physician in Sydney. For two years, he was medical columnist for the *Australian Women's Weekly*, and since 1990 he has been a Feldenkrais practitioner.

Lake has owned and run an art gallery which specialised in Australia-Pacific and pre-Columbian arts, and the work of contemporary local artisans; has written three books, including a volume of poetry; and has produced large numbers of scientific articles. His interests are classical music, painting, sculpture, writing, and permaculture. He swims summer and winter.

Bernard Lake believes that it is possible to slow the rate of ageing by adopting appropriate attitudes and behaviours. But, not surprisingly, he sees no chance of immortality.

I don't think anyone in their right mind would want to be immortal. What everybody wants is quality of life until it is time for exit, and it is really the last eighteen months or two years at the extreme end of life which is the most costly and disastrous. So far as we can tell at the moment, there is not much hope of reducing that kind of time.

At one stage, I was a physician at Lidcombe Hospital when it was an old man's home. The misery in the back blocks, where people didn't actually have any certifiable active disease, impressed me very deeply. I did a study which indicated that, at death, old men had at least four major conditions. You tend as you get older not to die from a specific disease—of course, the heart stops, so that could be called heart failure or whatever—but it impressed me that there was this continuous and insidious run-down in many of the systems of the body. Overall, there is a loss of water, and changes in the chemical bonds of many tissues; so my long suit since that time has been to determine what steps we could take to modify these changes. Long before it became fashionable, I was into the use of exercise regimes and modification of diet, trying to ensure that people got better sleep, that they kept themselves alive mentally as well as physically. Certainly, in my experience the people who have reached their eighties and nineties are people with tremendous spirit and go, who maintain an interest in what is going on around them.

*To what extent is there a biological clock in each person?*

Without doubt, if you are born into a family where your predecessors have all been long-lived, you have a better chance of also living to a great age; but no-one should sit around resting on their laurels because of that. For the people whose parents and grandparents have died at earlier ages, there are often a whole lot of social factors which are no longer operable—like changes in diet, smoking, and alcohol intake. There is the different incidence now for infectious diseases, and better medical support systems. So that, whilst genes set the overall pattern, statistically the variation is extraordinarily wide. Alternatively, if you are hell-bent or self-destructive, you can die as early as you like.

*Have you seen people who have been in extremely poor physical health and appearing to age rapidly, being able to turn that around?*

Oh, yes; this is part of the joy of my work. In 1967, I was inspired by a thoughtful businessman who wanted to increase his potential longevity and capacity. This was a strange thing to do at that time, but he opened my mind to all these possibilities. I had by the very nature of the practice to rely on simple expedients rather than various esoteric practices or drugs. On the other hand, where people need it, I will use everything I can lay my hands on to be of assistance to them. Whether it be orthodox or alternative is meaningless to me, as long as the measures are safe and effective.

*So when it comes to the whole ageing process, how important is it to work on all fronts: mind, body and spirit?*
It's essential to have a complex of things to work on. My aim is to help people to maximise themselves as human beings, and that requires careful and sometimes fairly strict attention to physical well-being. Then, for each individual to find what turns them on in terms of maintenance of interest in living; what will provide them with challenge that's not too threatening nor too great, but where there is interest in success and at completing each level of challenge.

*The degree to which we exercise appears to decline rapidly as we get older, so I would imagine you are often dealing with people where there is an ingrained resistance to change. How do you cope with that?*
Well, nature's implacable. If you haven't been exercising in your earlier years, you will lose your capacity for work output on a standardised test. You lose it at about 3 per cent per year after your maximum, which is actually in your thirties.

*[Laughter] There ain't much left in the end, is there?*
The good news is that, no matter at what age you start, even if it is seventy or eighty, you can get a percentage improvement on the baseline you began with. At that low level, every extra per cent of increase in your work capacity and your flexibility and co-ordination can lead to quite outstanding changes in your ability to look after yourself and to become plugged into life again.

*But do people mostly come when they are at a stage when they are almost dropping out of life? Are they at desperation point?*
My practice is widely drawn, because people only get referred to me if they have a problem. That problem may be one of anxiety when it

turns out they don't have a specific physical condition like cancer or heart disease. But they have major problems, or I would not be seeing them. I use that as an opportunity to ground them—perhaps for the first time—in a vision of what life could offer them overall. Most people make a positive choice. I also see quite a few people who decide to continue as before; and though I don't have any exact statistics, I can tell you that if you don't make the right choice then you have got to bear the consequences of increased ill-health and death.

*How does that affect you?*
I guess when I was younger I was so full of all the possibilities, I was perhaps over-enthusiastic. As I have got older I've realised that people have to make their own decisions. I can only give them the opportunity.

*Do you think that wisdom comes with age?*
I think wisdom is present right from childhood. Kids often say the most remarkable things, but they get told to shut up, or it's too embarrassing, because they have that beautiful naiveté that sees things very clearly. I think we spend most of the middle years of our life running away from wisdom, and we come back to wisdom as we get older and more certain of ourselves as individuals.

*That's interesting, because a couple of weeks ago I was with a Tibetan master, Sogyal Rinpoche, who was talking about the clutter of our minds—which are words I've heard you use. So it seems that we almost have to get rid of the clutter in order to get back to our innate selves?*
I couldn't agree with you more. So much of our life is lived on a superficial and trivial level. It's the way we deal with the trivia that is so important. If we allow them to grow like weeds, they'll be rampant and there's no way of getting rid of them. If we decide to cultivate our mental garden in a different way, the weeds have their place, but the other more positive plants flower as well.

*Why do we do that, I wonder?*
I think there is a social imperative for most people. In our society, which is very materialistic, you have got to have a bigger house, a better car. An enormous amount of social interaction occurs if you are involved in organisations which demand a kind of superficial compliance,

and that becomes impressed on your personality. So many people I know, including myself, have been through this. You have to be a professional, and you act as a professional, but your private life is something else. The trouble for most people is that they don't really have the time, opportunity, or know-how to quiet themselves sufficiently to really find out what their private life can offer them.

*So is this one of the bonuses of getting older: that either voluntarily or involuntarily some of the heat of work drops away, and there is more stillness and more peace?*
So many of the people that I know feel that each year has been getting better. I personally feel that, too. I realise what a crazy, mixed-up kid I was and probably still am, but I've managed to off-load—and so have they—a great deal of this excess clutter.

*How important are cultural and social attitudes to the ageing process?*
In strict and rigid communities they are very important. In a more open community like ours, I don't think they matter so much. What I think is terribly important is that interaction is available at all ages of existence, so that older people and younger people can talk freely together, and out of the ferment each can understand the other. I think in the more culturally rigid ethnic groups, to be aged means to be respected, because it means you have produced a brood of people that you have helped and then, in turn, they will look after you until death. Of course, that rigidity is being exploded as individualism comes more and more into the social fabric. When I was young, to be sixty was to be old. I'm sixty-four and I feel very youthful. I know that I'm also ageing. Very much so. I am very aware, because of friends and relatives and patients, that we are all ageing. But my spirit feels youthful and a hell of a lot freer than it did when I was younger.

*What happens to the brain in the ageing process?*
Well, that's an enormous question. In general, the brain remains as active as it was when it was younger if it's given the opportunity. Now, that opportunity may be compromised by changes in blood supply, and the same process of what is called atherosclerosis that affects the coronary arteries. It can be affected by all sorts of drugs and external toxins, pollutants, and goodness knows what else. But the brain is also informed by the body. It's wrong to think of the brain and the nervous

system as a unit. It's totally inextricably linked to what else is going on in the body and the information that is being fed through it. So it is more likely that you will have an active brain if you are an active person. That's not absolute—one only has to think of Stephen Hawking—but in general that is so.

As a follow-on from that activity, your arteries are more likely to be unclogged, and therefore blood distribution and all the glucose and nutrients necessary to sustain cells in action will continue. What is terribly important in the nervous system after birth, and through maturity and in later years, is that you keep on maintaining the web of connections which are made in the cells through what are called dendrites. You don't have any more cells when you die than you were born with, but you have an enormously increased number of connections. The more active your brain is, the more those connections are likely to multiply, and these seem to be the substrate of intelligent and purposeful activity as far as behaviour is concerned.

Mind and brain have been the subject of eternal disputes, but for simplicity I take mind as the evident operating apparatus of the brain at more subtle levels. There is no doubt that if you are well preserved physically, and if you continue to be 'in' life and not withdrawn from it, then the number of connections of these dendrites in your nervous system and your brain is substantial. You will have all your marbles and be able to continue.

Of course, there are very real potential problems. They cause various sorts of mental deterioration, such as Alzheimer's and certain kinds of Parkinson's disease, and so forth. The basic cause of these is subject to intensive research at the moment; I am not saying that we can all avoid those situations. One of the things that is very important is that it doesn't become so rich that it is overwhelming. In other words, within your brain and mind there is the opportunity to select what you are going to be interested in, how you are going to use that interest, and how you are going to link the richness within you—because if you make no effort to do that, you become more or less a passive receptor and increasingly disorganised.

I feel that this is what happens to many older people who are noted by their families to be a bit 'off'. They have chosen to withdraw and not expose this richness, not to use it. So this is why I am on about creating and maintaining challenge and interest according to individual design and motivation. I think that is extremely important. And to keep reviewing what is really essential in life, so we don't become overloaded.

*I'd like to talk about your childhood. Did you grow up with old people? Did your parents grow old well? Did you have positive role-models?*

My family was very ebullient. We were all very selfish kids; our parents thought the world of us, but they were also extremely encouraging. They both came from poor, hard, working-class backgrounds. They wanted only that we did better than they had done. We had nothing but encouragement from them, and a lot of direction which was almost indirect. My father was extraordinarily hard working, and my mother coped with us somehow—which was extremely hard—to the best of her ability.

*What did your father do?*

He was in the film business. He ran away from home, and he entered the AIF when he was sixteen—below age—and he was demobilised in France at the end of the war. He went to England and then to America. He worked in a steel foundry for about six years and was doing very well there, but he met up with a buddy from the war who said the motion picture industry is really where it is all at. So he got into the motion picture industry in America, and then came back here. He was the general sales manager at MGM, which was then of course the mighty company. So we had a very privileged existence. Hopefully, all of us made the most of that. My brother Max became a surgeon; my brother Jeff—who has just died—was a dentist; and my sister went into education.

*This sounds like four people who were very high-achieving. Were you ambitious?*

I don't think that we felt particularly ambitious at all; it was just in the milieu that was created by my parents. My father loved knowledge, and we were always being subject to bits of information and encyclopedias and God knows what else, and it was just fun to be able to talk about what was going on in the world and what interested us. Both parents showed great interest in whatever interested us. For them, I guess, it was a creative education; it was the feedback. So there was a kind of ferment in the house the whole time. I don't think we measured ourselves against what was going on outside.

*Did your parents live a long time?*
No. My father died in his fifties from a coronary heart attack, and mum died in her early seventies. One of my everlasting regrets is that both of them, as I know now, could have lived a hell of a lot longer.

*Has this influenced you at all do you think?*
Oh, I would think, in a deep way, yes. Not too consciously, but certainly we boys were conscious of trying to make our mid-fifties, and get beyond it.

*How strong are some of those experiences that we bring from childhood to the way we cope with getting older?*
Wow, that's a question. Well, I think it is very difficult, because we are all subject to the family milieu. And, as I say, we were very privileged to have such an upbringing. So because of this encouragement of our curiosity, and our personal further reaching to do whatever we felt we were capable of, we were never denied. There were times when the parents were horrified at what we were trying to do or wanted to do. For instance, I put a pack on my back when I was fifteen, and said, 'These holidays, I'm going hitchhiking.' And they spent many sleepless nights when I was hitchhiking. It was a magnificent experience. That kind of thing, the freedom and the trust, I've always been grateful for it. As a kind of quid pro quo, whenever I wanted to be a biologist, the folks leaned hard on me to become a medico as a more suitable compromise. And so it came to pass.

On the other hand, within my own later life, I've had a hell of a lot of fascinating experiences which added to my sense of personal richness of what life has to offer. When I was a teenager, I had my first mystical experience, which was just absolutely astounding. It knocked me for a long time. I thought who in the world can I share this with. I couldn't share it with my parents—they wouldn't understand it. I couldn't share it with anyone. That set me off on a path of search. People do have these experiences, and they are shattering, and they are profoundly life-directing. So that's been out of the family—quite separate—and very much orienting my whole attitude to life and how to live it.

*Can you describe the experience?*
I was out bushwalking with a friend. We were in the Blue Mountains, and it was raining like hell. We were exhausted, and we finally found a

little cave in the side of the mountain where we could shelter. My friend fell asleep immediately, and I just sat at the mouth of the cave looking at the storm, which was quite spectacular—the changes in the cloud and the wind patterns. Then the clouds began to lift, and suddenly I saw this object in the sky: it got larger and larger, and I suddenly realised it was actually two eagles doing a mating wheeling. The eagles lock their talons together and cartwheel on the airlifts. Something happened at that time, and I don't know how long I was there, but I just felt completely at one with the universe—well, I lost the ego—and I felt so privileged to be part of this whole deal.

*What interests me is how these quite extraordinary moments then leave us. I guess we carry the awareness within us, but why do they go? Do you think that we could have them more readily available?*

Yes. It takes a lifetime to find out how [laughter]. In recent years, I am particularly keen on what I call being 'present'. That means that you are totally with the now, and that's a very big deal for most of us, including myself. By being totally present you are really in the stream of your being with whatever the great being is—the total universe. If you can achieve that, it doesn't matter what you do in life: from sitting on the toilet, washing up the dishes, being by yourself, being with friends, there is a totally new dimension to that whole interchange. It doesn't mean that you withdraw from life; it just means that you are fully into life, and every moment counts. I think that this has also become commonplace. Carlos Castaneda in his books always speaks about Don Juan saying something like, 'Death should always be present on your shoulder.' And the meaning of that to me is that death being—as far as we know—our ultimate finality, this carries such an imprint that, if we died right now, would this have been our greatest moment? Most of us can truthfully say, 'No way!' On the other hand, once you begin to get this sense of the general pulse of the universe, you can more truthfully say, 'Perhaps this is the best moment.'

*For you, then, is there an ultimate finality? Or do you feel the essence of you will continue in some way?*

The answer for me is that death is final. The only essence that will continue to exist will be imprinted on the brains of people I have known, and whenever they choose to think of me some part of that interaction will, of course, be revived. But, beyond that, I don't think so. I think this is why people become artists, and should become artists. Because wherever art survives it has the opportunity to imprint something of your personal magic on other people, and for those other people to begin to interact. One of my great moments was being in the National Gallery in London. I had been wandering around for the afternoon when I was suddenly caught by this portrait—it turned out to be by Rembrandt—and I was absolutely seized by the magic of the personality that was shining out of this picture which was painted three hundred and fifty years before. That particular set of circumstances that brought me to the gallery, that particular portrait that caught me, brought me in touch with Rembrandt and what this guy was on about, and why people had raved about him. And so Rembrandt lived for me, as do great composers and musicians. But it would be the ultimate selfishness to believe that any other than some kind of fragmentary part of us is likely to be 'eternal'. I personally can't feel that.

*Do you sense any kind of meaning to life? Or is the meaning of life, life itself?*

Absolutely, yes, it's totally that. That's why it's so important for all of us to be really in touch with this stream of being—so that, if we do die right at this next moment, we will have really got the most out of existence, and given the most to existence. So many of us dodge those issues. That's okay; I feel quite at ease about people making their own decisions about this. I'm just talking personally.

*Do you fear dying?*

I did. I don't fear it any more. I would like to die peacefully and without too much pain. But I know it's inevitable; and, as you get older, one of the things that certainly brings you wisdom, if you are prepared for it, is the death of friends, relatives, acquaintances and, of course, patients—and recognising each time the possibility for re-ordering your own existence in a more seemly fashion for yourself.

*Do you think that people should be able to end their lives when they choose?*

Sure. I have no problems with this at all. I'll tell you a little story: when I was a young intern working in London, I spent the whole of one Saturday sitting at the bedside of a woman who had been admitted with a possible endocrine disorder. She was hirsute, large, and very distressed. She came from an English family, but had been brought up in India. Her parents had died. She was friendless. She was living in a little room in Hampstead all by herself; she had no-one to talk to, and was utterly depressed. And the likelihood of making effective human contact was very limited.

So as a keen young guy I sat there, and we talked for hours. I left her only when she promised me—she was talking suicide the whole time—that suicide was out of the question. She had actually begun to smile, and we cracked a few jokes. I walked out feeling, wow, I had done a marvellous job. About two hours after, she suddenly leapt out of bed, got herself dressed, raced down to the Hampstead tube, and threw herself under a train. If people are bent on suicide, they will suicide. Most people are not bent on suicide. They are desperate, and they need help, and they need people-contact of a kind that hasn't been forthcoming. Many kids attempt suicide in the desperate hope that, in being found and helped, this will tide them over into a better kind of life.

*It has often seemed paradoxical to me that our increasing technological knowledge enables us to live longer; and yet with that we seem to have lost touch with ourselves, with a lot of our sensory perceptions.*

The best of technology has been an undeniably magnificent aid to human beings in the West. Things like hip replacements—people who would slowly die and perish because of their immobility in all sorts of nasty ways—are up and mobile. There are all sorts of developments in medicine and in technology which are very helpful to maintaining the aged in comfort. We are all aware of the bad sides of technology, and that's no different to the downsides of us as human beings. We are all wonderful people; we are also dreadful people, all of us. We all share that spectrum; not one of us is free from it. It depends where you make your individual choice in that spectrum as to how you appear to yourself and how you appear to other people.

We have that choice as the overall begetters of technology, to order our technology in such ways to protect the environment, and to make cities more cheerful and more livable. Of course, we don't make those choices, except small bands of people within a community may have very strong views one way or another. In order to convince other members of the community, they often go overboard in presenting these views. It is very difficult at any time to get human beings to be consensual; it's almost impossible, but it can be done. There are always individuals who come at a time and circumstance, and are charismatic enough, to carry the day. Like the man who decided to clean up Sydney, and it's now the world. I read somewhere recently that there are up to thirty million people participating in this one-day gesture of trying to clean up the world. Okay, perhaps that's just a drop in the ocean; but it does show there are these possibilities for human beings to make a gesture that will be really significant. If the critical mass is achieved, then that becomes the next social imperative.

*Are things improving, or are we forever in a cyclical stage of one step forward, one step back?*

I don't see it as cyclical, I see it as paradoxical. The point is, when is the paradox going to burst? Soon there will be five-and-a-half billion people on the face of the earth, perhaps two-thirds of whom will not have enough to eat, and a majority of the kids will die from starvation and disease. I don't believe in the Micawber kind of thing—that everything is going to turn out for the best—at all. I think we have more responsible decisions to make about how we are going to nurture the earth than we have ever had in our existence; and if we don't make the right decisions and take the appropriate actions, then Gaia will do the job. We are just one of millions of possible species on the face of the earth. If all humanity is blotted out within a geological time-frame, something else will happen, and new species will emerge. But somewhere in the universe there will be a black mark that we haven't made the right choices.

*Do you feel optimistic or pessimistic?*

All this is going to come to more obvious conclusions after I'm gone. I'm certainly doing my damnedest in my own small way to be on the side of maintaining the earth as a habitable place. But I won't be making the ultimate decisions, although I feel very strongly that those decisions should be taken now before there is an inevitability which is obviously unavoidable in twenty or thirty years' time.

*As short as that, do you feel?*

Sure. Things are already changing. We are losing our corals around the world; all sorts of indications are there. And we can keep on turning a blind eye and saying, 'Oh well, that's just another freak of nature; corals were meant to die out.' Well, human beings were meant to die out as well, surely. We are aware of presiding over the extinction of many other plants and animals. This is ridiculous. If we look at all the bits of information that are now available to us, we have to take decisions, right around the world, right through every government, about how we are going to manage this earth responsibly.

*How would you like to be remembered?*
How would I like to be remembered? Well, frankly, it doesn't matter what I feel about that [laughter] I will be remembered by those who choose to remember me. My hope is that, among my intimates, they'll have a nice warm and loving feeling, and feel that I've been of some help, or provided them with some pleasure or joy in their life-path.

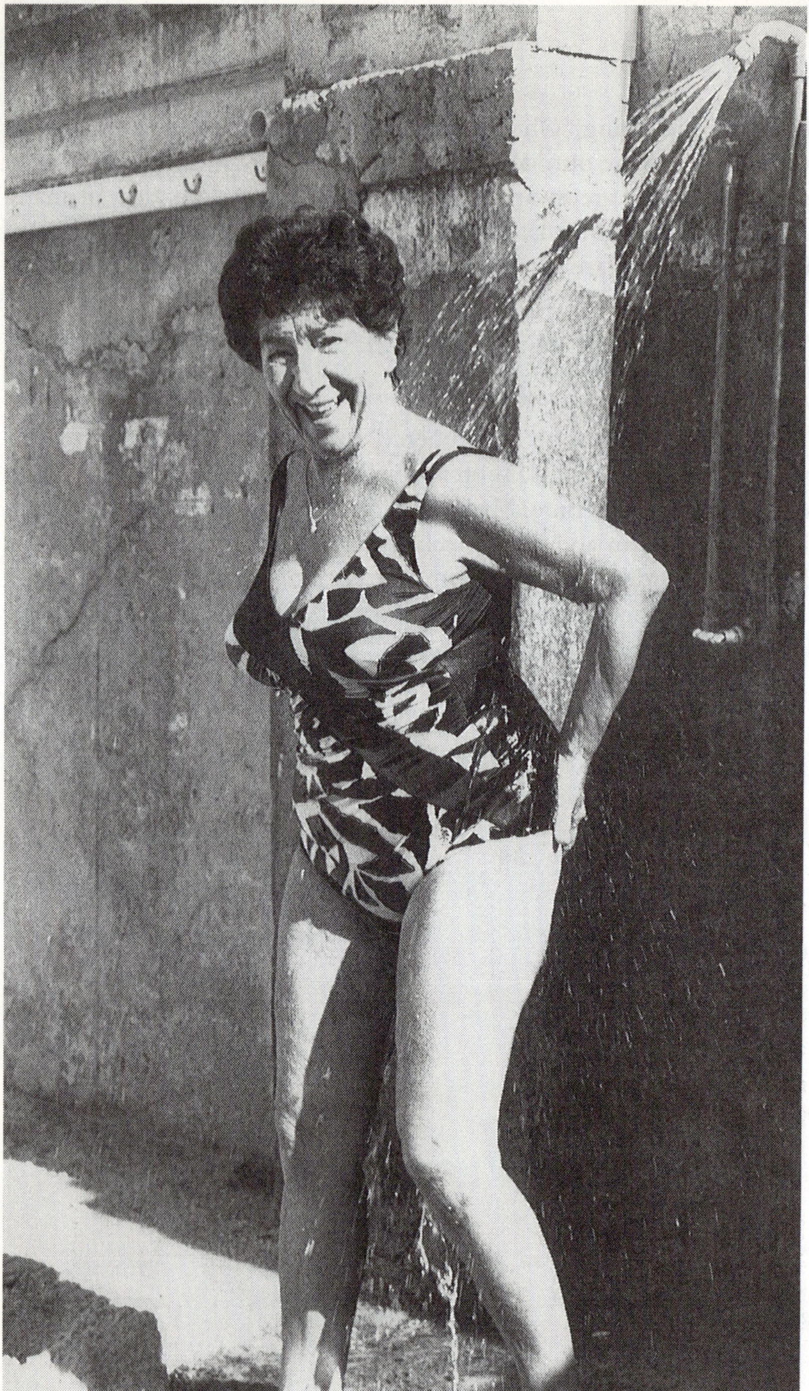

# Dorothy Buckland-Fuller
*The wise ones*

Dorothy Buckland-Fuller was born Dorothea Dimitropoulou in Port Said on 21 January 1922 of Greek parents. Her father was a businessman who also worked for the Greek church. She says they were not rich, but they were not poor. She worked in London with the BBC, and then with Niarchos, the Greek millionaire, before coming to Australia with her family in 1961 because of problems in Egypt.

One of her first jobs was as secretary to the production manager of a big clothing company; buyers complained about her accent, and she was fired. She told her story to an ABC current affairs program, and letters in her support came flooding in. This was her first encounter with racism in Australia, and it led to her life-time involvement helping ethnic communities achieve justice. She studied sociology at the University of New South Wales so that she would be well equipped for her campaigns, and has served on a large number of ethnic affairs bodies, including the Ethnic Affairs Commission of NSW. She is also a member of the NSW Consumer Forum for the Aged.

Dorothy Buckland-Fuller lectures, produces a multitude of publications, and doesn't give any indication of slowing down. She lives in an apartment in Balmoral, practices Tai Chi, swims and walks on the beach all year round, and says she never tries to hide her age.

I tell people about my age because it is very important especially to tell women that I am over seventy. They don't believe it, my students don't believe it and, when I am leading the Greek dancing, nobody believes it [chuckles].

*Why do you think it's important?*
Because a great number of people think that when they grow old they're finished, especially women—you know, men want younger women. Why should we care what men want or not if we enjoy life? I enjoy life to the full. Every minute I do something useful and enjoyable. Sometimes I do useful things that I don't enjoy, but not very often. I do a lot of community work; then you lose yourself in the whole, and you feel that your life has meaning. Otherwise, life is meaningless. I am here, I produced a daughter, I have a house or a flat or a unit or something, and then what! So, I have a lot of love, I have a great number of friends, and there's a lot of cuddles and kissing.

Every two months we go to this taverna which is called Scorpio's and we do Greek dancing. This is my way of seeing my friends, because I have so many—we had seventy people once—and as they arrive we cuddle and I introduce them to each other, which is good. Positive energy and happiness are contagious. I have found out that when I am with people even angry feelings are transformed into loving and positive feelings. This is my religion. This is what I believe.

*Have you always been like this?*
More and more. I was a happy person. I come from a family of six. My grandmother used to live nearby, so it was a big household with lots of noise and laughter. My parents were happy, loving each other. My family here is very caring. I never ask them for anything, but I know they're there if I need them. I have a daughter, too, but I never ask her either. I am very independent.

*Do you think there is a special role for older people?*
Yes, we should be the peacemakers, the love-spreading ones, if we can use words like this, to pass round to other people the knowledge that they can be happy without material things. Definitely people need their bread and butter and their roof over their head, but we can share. There is so much in this country we could all be wealthy. But that is not enough. If I had to lose what I have here in my home, or to keep

the love of my friends, I'd choose the love of my friends.

Old people should be respected and honoured as 'The Wise Ones.' They should be given the opportunity to contribute what they know, and to share that knowledge with other people, provided they are not selfish. Some people, as they grow old, they want to hold on to everything—to positions of power, to material things. If people come here and they like something, unless it has a special sentimental value for me, I say, 'Take it.'

*What is Australia like in terms of its attitude to old people?*
Well, I'm afraid that in Australia—and it's becoming so in Europe—when you are very young you are brought up to stress individualism and separateness. You call it 'independence.' I call it 'separateness.' It starts from a very early age when there is separation between the older people and the young people. In Greek culture they grow up together, all the generations; so young children, they get used to older skin, and older people to be around, so they don't see them as different. There is an affinity between grandparents and grandchildren, much more than between parents and children, because the parents have the hassles to keep the kids in order. The grandparents have to look after them very often, but they have more time and they have the philosophy and the patience. The older women are the confidantes and the matchmakers. They know about herbs, about everything. Back home, they used to act as midwives. I learned so many things from the villagers. I love going to Greece and talking with the older women. Older men are okay, but it is the women as a rule who are the wise ones.

In Australia, I have found that the older people are seen as old fashioned, passé, finished, and we use the word 'aged.' I refuse to use this word. I say 'ageing'. Ageing is a process. I am ageing from the moment I am born; whereas 'aged' is a past tense, something finite. I don't feel one day older than when I was in my twenties. I see my wrinkles, and then what! They are irrelevant. I will use a cream mainly to clean my face, but I don't spend time, I never go to beauticians; I cut my own hair. All these things I do myself, because I think they are important, but not my priority.

I have found out that, wherever I go, it is very important for me to say the things I say, especially to Anglo-Saxon friends, and especially to young people. For example, if I give a lecture on ageing and the different way the ethnic communities treat older people, the students like it. So

I say to them, 'Just think that one day you, too, are going to be old, and the type of society that we help to develop now is the society into which we will all grow old.' It's funny when I say, 'I will grow old.' People say, 'At seventy-two, she *is* old!' [laughs]

Psychologists talk now about skin hunger, when the skin of people needs to be hugged; and skin deprivation, when they don't get the hugs. Nowadays they have to bring dogs into nursing homes so the older people can touch the animal, because they don't have humans to touch. I think that's very sad. I am sure these older people would rather have had their grandchildren. There was that case recently of a woman in her seventies or eighties, who was found to have been dead for three months and nobody knew she had died. This is terrible.

**There are also very strong cultural attitudes towards women getting old which can be oppressive.**

The same thing applies in Europe. Men want younger women, much younger. The men are sixty and they look seventy, and they want a woman of forty—which is ridiculous. And if they meet a woman of sixty or seventy they say she is too old for them. But they're okay at the age of sixty or seventy. That's generally, although now here in Australia there is a reversal. Some women, they do marry younger men or they go out with younger men; which is a good thing, because of these attitudes.

In Western societies, women are losing power as they grow older because they lose their looks; whereas in traditional societies—in Greece, for example, especially in the small towns and villages—the woman's power is growing with age, and we still find older women who are honoured by their children and grandchildren. When I go to the villages, I see the women outside their door talking with each other, knitting or shelling peas or doing something. They are never alone because of their neighbourhood.

Here, people lock themselves in their homes—their castles! Even in the ethnic communities, people nowadays live far away from each other. Some of them choose to remain in small areas, some move out to more prestigious suburbs, and they lose out in the process, because they're locked away in big homes. They're wealthy but when they grow old they live alone, and it's very sad. I still think I would rather spend my last years in Greece, and die on a small island —but I can't because of my family being here. The kids respect old people. They kiss their hands to show affection and respect.

Here, I've noticed things are changing a little bit, but before it was awful—the patronising way in which some nurses used to pat older people on the head like children. I *cuddle*, and there is a difference. You put your arms around them and you touch them. I stroke people all the time on the face.

*It's quite true that business about children sometimes being frightened of old people, because the smell or the touch is strange.*
That's terrible! Ten years ago, I was running a seminar in Sweden—they have secondary school children going as part of their school work to older people's homes and helping them with their grooming, bathing, etc, so children get used to old skin from a very young age. I have told people about that at various meetings here, and nobody listens.

*Do you ever get tired?*
No, no. I am never tired. Well, no, I am very rarely tired. I get tired when I am emotionally upset about other people's problems, when there is nothing I can do to help. I have lots of energy, but sometimes—like last week—I was involved with a project about women who were retrenched, and you feel all the pain and the depression and the negative energy in them, and you take it on you. And then when I came home, I was tired. But I had a shower [chuckles], and I just thought of something positive. I said, 'Well, I helped. I gave them some hope.' Not only hope, but we gave them addresses where they could go and find assistance. I believe that it is not enough helping only one person, and that is why I am concentrating mainly on issues—so we can change attitudes, we can change policies.

*Are you a very organised person?*
[Laughter] I am the most disorganised person in the whole world. I just let things happen. I do one thing at a time as it comes my way. You, Anne, are here now, and you are the most important person this minute. The past is gone. The future might never come. I might die tonight. I am not scared of death, either, but I would like to be able to choose when I die. When I am ready I would like to will it, and go to bed and sleep and never to wake up. If not, I believe in voluntary euthanasia. I believe by the time I am ready, before I lose my dignity and self-respect, I will be able to take a tablet and go to sleep. I think it

is a terrible thing what they are doing here to people, keeping them alive when they wish to be free from pain and self-pity. A person like me staying in bed for ever! I wouldn't like to be a burden on society or my family.

I am a coward. I don't like to have pain, and I don't like taking tablets, not even aspirins. If I'm sick I might take antibiotics, but I prefer to go through unwell spells without any drugs of any type, because I think they fix one thing and they mess up something else. I watch what I eat. I am very careful. I wash things very well because of all the poisons. I soap all fruit; I rinse it well. I rinse all the dishes. I don't allow these terrible chemicals they put on things to enter my body. Maybe that's part of my energy. Maybe it's my love of people; maybe it's my Tai Chi; maybe it's my swimming; maybe it's a combination of everything. I don't know.

*Do you look back on your life very much?*

Very rarely. Only when I am talking with people and things come up, but I haven't got time to sit down and think what happened in the past. When I am talking with people I think of past things sometimes, and I bring them up if they are useful. Otherwise, to reminisce and feel sorry, no.

*Has sex and sexuality got a role to play in the life of old people?*

I think yes. It depends how you define sexuality. You see, people think it's the sex act. For me, it's cuddling and stroking; and maybe the way I compensate, because I live by myself, is all these lovely people that I cuddle, the young ones, the older ones, everybody, all the people I have this affection for. And all my other activities. People need love, need the touching. We need to feel another human being. That's why, as I say, people resort to animals, and that's okay.

I wouldn't mind if in this block there were friends of mine next door and below, and in our old age we could share by each one being independent in our own unit, but meeting when we need. You need intelligent people who don't become pests. I respect other people's space, and I expect other people to respect mine. I need my peace and quiet, and the only way I get it—because my telephone is going all the time—is by going off every now and then to Greece. I don't plan; I never book when I go anywhere. I find a village, I ask a taxi driver to find a woman who is a widow and she lives on her own and has a room to spare, and I go there. You learn about the people of the country and you talk to them on a one-to-one basis, as a woman towards another woman.

*You obviously travel light?*
Oh yes, a very small bag—the bag that people take when they go, let's say, from here to Woollongong. Because, you see, if I need anything I can buy it. Why cart things with me? I take a spare pair of shoes, a couple of pieces of underwear, a couple of dresses, my bathing costume, and sometimes a jacket [chuckles]

*Dorothy, you talked briefly about older people in your childhood. What are some of those memories?*
My grandmother used to always yell at us when she really loved us. I used to say she was laughing under her moustache—that's a Greek expression. She was a very fierce-looking, very strong woman, but she loved us and I could feel this. She was smiling while telling us off, chasing us but laughing. I remember my father and mother loving each other. They never displayed love by kissing in public—couples, you know, you see them, 'Darling, kiss-kiss' and then God knows what! No, but I could see it. Sometimes, for example, my mother would take some water to my father because, at the end of his life, he was blind. And when she went near him, she would just touch his arm. You don't have to display love; you can see it in the eyes.

I believe a lot in body language. When I go like this and stroke people, it's because I care for people. I had three brothers and two sisters. One of my brothers died, so we were five children at the end, and there was a lot of love, and no jealousy. All these psychologists with their theories on sibling rivalry! I am also concerned to hear so many young women who are against the mother. I loved my mother and I loved my grandmother. I liked to go out, and they used to yell at me. I fought with them, but I never hated them.

I was never jealous of my sisters who were younger and prettier. I loved my sisters and they loved me. I have never come across a Greek woman of my generation who hated her mother—and I asked a great many of them. But that's how people are brought up nowadays: to believe that all the things wrong in their life are the fault of their parents, and I disagree. I've been thinking of writing a book in defence of mothers [laughter].

*Do you think we still are a racist country?*
Yes, we are a racist country. Even the ethnic communities who have experienced racism and know how it hurts, they are racist towards the newcomers, the Asian people; and we are all racist towards the Aborigines. I think it's a terrible thing. I was appalled when I first came to Australia in 1961, to find out the way people were talking about Aborigines, as if they were nothing, rubbish, drunkards. And then, when I started learning more about it, I felt ashamed of all of us Europeans. After I lost my job because of my accent, I decided to study at the University, to work with the ethnic communities to balance the injustice a bit, and I became very much involved with ethnic affairs.

*Where do you think this comes from, this drive to leave the world a better place? Your parents?*
[Laughter] No. On the contrary, my family thinks I am crazy. They keep on saying, 'Why on earth you spend so much time doing all these things without getting paid?' But I just feel like it. I think that if each one of us does not put our little stone to this monument that we want to call civilisation, there will be no civilisation. We must not allow the forces of destruction and of evil to go ahead. I am concerned at the destruction of the environment, the arms trade, the gambling casinos, racist groups, and the computer taking over our lives. I believe that all thinking, caring people should do something to make this a better society.

For me, Australia could become the lighthouse of the world. We have every ethnic group practically from every part of the world, and it could be a harmonious, prosperous society if we were less greedy. I have friends who have so much, they don't know what they have; and yet they are so insensitive to other people's needs. Well, I can't. I have some friends who are real capitalists. They say, 'Dorothy, you too are a capitalist: you own a place, you have a car, etc.' I say, 'Yes, but if I give them away, what do I do?' Whereas by keeping them and by educating myself I can fight in a voluntary capacity. All my paid work is five hours, enough for my bread and butter; the rest of my time I give doing things to improve our society and to help other people. This is my way to give meaning to my life.

*You spoke about having a spiritual feeling, one of belonging. Would you talk about that a little?*

I would define myself as a non-religious person. I don't say atheist, because that has certain connotations as if there is or isn't a God. I say that my mind and everybody else's is not big enough to grasp the enormity of what is around us. I think it is as arrogant to say there is a God, and God is a male white Anglo-Saxon or Greek Orthodox or whatever [laughs] as it is to say there is nothing. All I know is that there is an energy which I feel with people. I've read quite a lot about other religions. Basically, all religions and all philosophies boil down to the same rules: be kind to your neighbour; don't do unto other people what you don't want them to do unto you; and give love.

*Do you think ahead?*

No, I just live one day at a time. I do have an idea of what I would like the future to be, and if I had power what I would be doing. But if I were to think all the time of these things, I wouldn't be doing all the other things I am doing, and I am a doer.

*If you had power, what would you be doing?*

My taxation system would be very different to the taxation system as it is now. I would include in education a philosophy of life that means sharing things with people, developing neighbourhoods—small neighbourhoods where people can help each other. Teach at school less greed. You see, we tell people how important it is to 'make it', and 'making it' means having material things. But at the end of the count we all have two yards of soil to go into, and you need nothing. Teach people and give them the feeling of what it means to love and to be loved. To be loved you have to love, and to be loved you have to be unselfish and to get rid of the capital 'E' in front of your ego. We all have egos, we can't live without them; but reduce them. Teach children from very young how to share. My students are encouraged to share everything. They can do collective essays, collective everything, and because they are doing it together it's easier, better and it's more fun.

*What would you do as far as old people are concerned?*

I wouldn't isolate them. I like the idea of granny flats. Every person who has a house should have a smaller place at the back for the grandmothers, so they'll be close but at the same time have their privacy. I would educate the young people to use but not abuse their grandmothers. Because right now with the ethnic communities, for example, the grandmother is used a lot to look after the kids when they are little; but then when they grow up neither the children nor the grandchildren want her around. They see her as old fashioned and interfering, and there are arguments and harsh words. They wouldn't dare to do that back in the village, because of the shame and the dishonour it would bring to them. But nobody knows them here, so they can neglect or even send the older people into a nursing home. I think nursing homes should be the last resort, when the family cannot cope any more and we would have two sick people instead of one.

There should be much more help. Home care, for example, should become more effective. Staff should get more training in sensitivity and understanding. There is also a question of courtesy and good manners. Older people have been brought up to respect and consider others, and feel hurt when they are treated casually. I think there should be much more emphasis on how to behave towards old people. What's the use of me having assistance for home care or for another service when it's done without affection or respect, and when the staff treat me in a patronising way? This is counter-productive, because it affects the emotional well-being of older people.

I think we should have older people in positions of power in service-providing organisations, because they've experienced life. In fact, there should be an older person and a younger person in every job; one job could be quite well shared between two, sometimes three, people. We could all lower our material expectations and be happier with less pay and fewer hours, and have more time to enjoy life. People don't realise how lovely it is not to have to work full-time. I put my five hours in one day at the University, and the rest of the time I do voluntary work—which means I don't feel the obligation to be there. I do have the obligation, but if I can't and I don't feel well, I won't go. I ring and say, 'I'm sorry I can't come.' If I don't have the time to read all the minutes and all the papers, well, I just go there and I listen. I don't participate. You see, it's important to realise the benefits of freedom. I can go for a walk, I can do whatever I like, get up any time I like, go to bed late. Before, if I went to bed late, I was thinking, 'Oh, I have to get up early in the morning.' Now I go to bed and I say, 'Well if I don't wake up, that's it!' So it's beautiful.

It's important for people to understand that you can learn so many things. Twelve years ago, I went to a summer school and decided to learn pottery; so I began making pots and I thought, 'Isn't that lovely!'

I couldn't draw a straight line, so one year I went to a painting class and discovered that I could paint. Now I paint, I do pottery, and if I can't sleep at night—not very often—I get up and I start painting all over my existing paintings. If you look at the paintings around my flat, maybe they have been painted over many times. They change with my mood.

Life can be so much fun. I am not rich, but I am not very poor. I can do all these things, and I am lucky to have the aptitude and attitude towards doing them. But there are some people who never had the chance. I was talking earlier about all these women who have been retrenched. One of them said, 'For thirty years I haven't been out of my home and the factory.' They don't know the world. They haven't got a clue what's going on out there. It's easy and arrogant for me to talk like this, but we should give opportunity to all the ageing people to taste these things. Instead of that we just dampen their enthusiasm.

*Bertrand Russell once said, 'Never try to suppress enthusiasm, you're bound to succeed.' Is there anything you would like to say to older people?*

I would like to say, 'Act your age but don't be ashamed to feel the life force in you. Do some dancing. Tell your children that you don't want to stay home and look after their kids all the time. One of them can stay home and look after the kids, and the other can take you to a Greek dance where you don't need a partner. Forget your feet and dance with your heart. Become very useful to yourself and others by joining groups or organisations. Grow all the time, learn something, go to the older people's centre, meet with other people, show your enthusiasm so you enthuse others also, because people—especially people of non-English-speaking background think, 'People will laugh at me.' Don't care about anybody laughing at you. If they want to laugh that is their problem.

Look after your health. Watch what you are eating but don't become fanatical; just enjoy every now and then what you like to enjoy. The most important thing is love. Meet with people, cuddle people. You have the opportunity to put your arms round anybody you like— young, old, anybody. I cuddle so many young people it's incredible. All the handsome young men that all the young girls would wish they could put their arms around, they say, 'Dorothy, how lucky you are.' And I say, 'Of course I am.' And they love me, they put their arms around me and they lift me up, some of my spiritual brothers and sons. And it's beautiful because they need a grandmother or a mother, and I need sons and daughters and grandsons and grand-daughters. These are beautiful relationships.

I would also like to say, 'Do something that makes you feel that your life has meaning.' I think the most important thing for me is to leave a better society to my daughter and nephews and nieces and all the children of the world that I see as my children; to leave a happier society not only in Australia, but to leave a happier world.

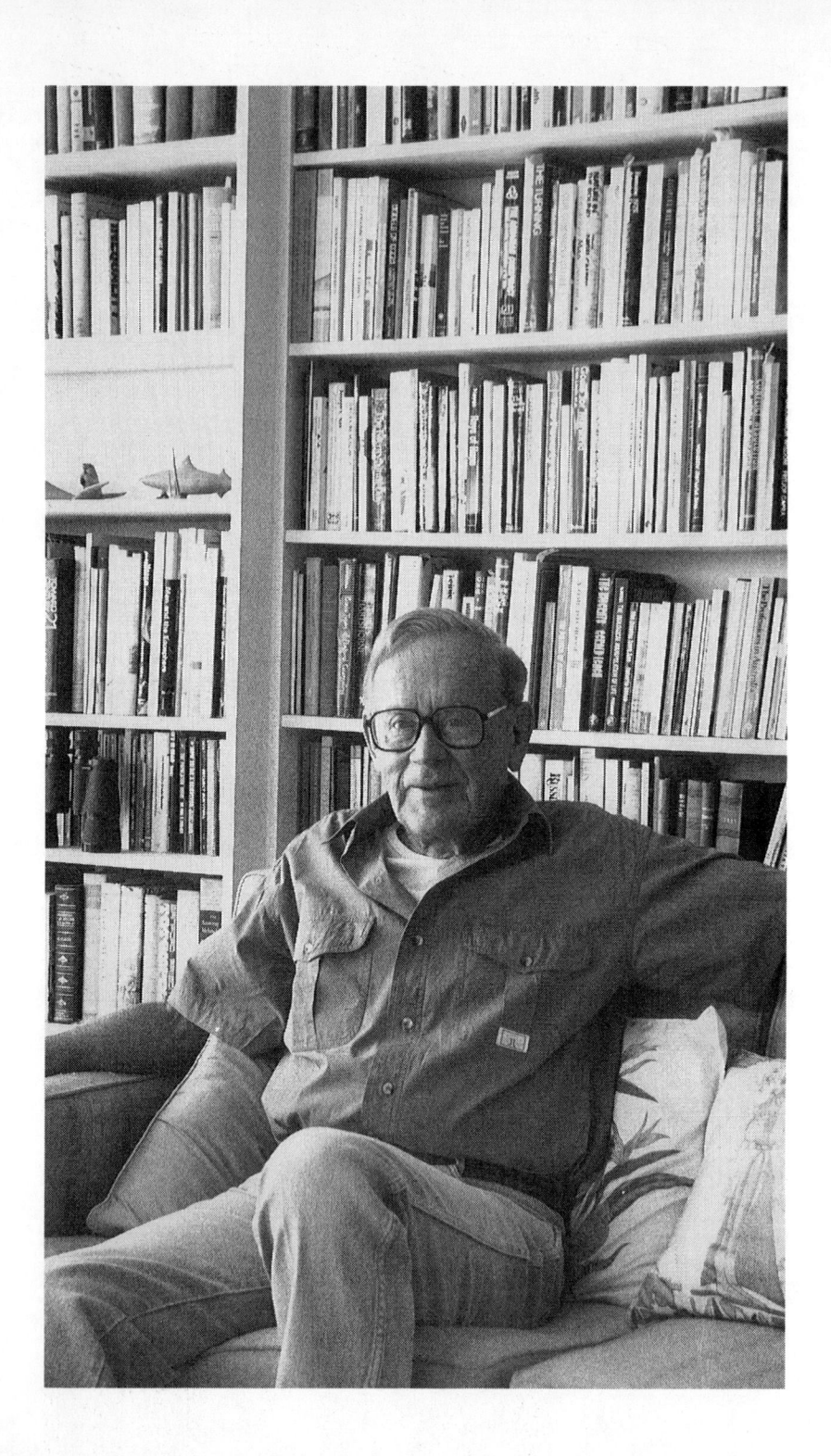

# Charles Birch
*It's important to be excited*

Charles Birch is a distinguished scientist, scholar, and Emeritus Professor of Science at the University of Sydney. His books raise fundamental issues concerning theology, science, and ecology, and his work has been recognised by the richest and most prestigious international prize 'for progress in religion', the Templeton Award. *Regaining Compassion* published in 1993, drew scientist Paul Ehrlich to comment that it was especially recommended to those who think that 'science has all of the answers'. Birch says that his book is about relating: 'relating to oneself, to others, to other living creatures, to the world and to God.'

Birch was born in Melbourne in February 1918, and studied at the Universities of Melbourne and Adelaide. From 1960 to 1984, he was Challis Professor of Biology at the University of Sydney. He has held visiting professorships at a number of overseas universities. He was one of the first and strongest voices to publicly question Australia's involvement in the war in Vietnam and, at the same time, he founded an organisation to assist Australian students who were refusing conscription. Later, he worked at the Wayside Chapel, helping homeless young people in Sydney's King's Cross.

He lives in a Sydney apartment overlooking the harbour. Throughout the interview he kept breaking away to feed birds that flew down to the terrace railings.

If I'm given invitations to talk, I prefer to accept those that involve young people. All my friends are about half my age. I suppose I feel that the oldies can't do as much to change the world, whereas the younger generation might—people who are thinking of the next step in their profession, and vastly enthusiastic at doing something about the environment. I feel excited about meeting people like that. I get the spirit of being young again, and how wonderful it is to have all those enthusiasms. I suppose they're interested in me because I've solved some problems that they haven't, and I'm interested in them because they're trying to solve problems. I have always been surrounded by students.

*When you were a young man did you think about age?*
Never thought about it at all. Just content to look up to men who were greying around their temples.

*So in your life, have there been older people who have influenced you?*
Every step of my life there have been older people who have influenced me. I think one of the important things is that if I hadn't had that influence I would have felt insecure. It took me a long time to really think I could do something on my own. Why did I have doubts? Oh, I don't think I had any reason to suppose I would be particularly good at an academic career.

*Did your parents have the same kind of intellectual curiosity and excitement that you have?*
Ah, yes, except my father was a bank manager. I don't think I gained much from him, but my mother was brought up in a convent in Dublin. She was a nursing sister. She was always curious in the sense of reading avidly, giving me lots of stuff to read—like books by J B S Haldane, Julian Huxley, and other biologists. She taught me never to pass a word without looking it up in the dictionary if I didn't understand it. She was rather traditional in her religious beliefs and feeling, and thought that I was getting a bit way out. But that didn't bother me too much.

I had two brothers, a twin brother and another older brother who was a pilot during the war; after the war he became a Qantas pilot. He was excited about flying. The other brother was a personnel officer with Shell. So both were quite different.

*At what stage in your life did you begin to be interested in spiritual concerns?*

When I was at school. I was at Scotch College in Melbourne, and the only religious influence there was a fairly strong evangelical outfit called the Crusader Movement which I now look back on with some horror. It was fundamentalist and very straight-laced. I suppose I thought, 'That's probably the truth. What alternative is there?'—and everybody said, 'There is no alternative.' When I went to University I got tied up with this same sort of fundamentalist movement, but more reluctantly. It wasn't until I became a graduate student, working on research, that I was challenged by my superiors on the funny ideas that I had. Fortunately, I then found another group, the Student Christian Movement, which was a very liberal organisation. You didn't have to sign on the dotted line or anything like that.

*In those days, did scientists tend to be cut off from spiritual issues—unlike today, where there is considerable interchange of ideas and beliefs?*

Certainly, that was true in the environment in which I lived. Pretty well everybody in the research institute in which I was involved was agnostic. We all talked to each other, it was quite a small laboratory, and they regarded religion as very unscientific. No, there certainly has been a change on the religious frontier, because the scientific, technological world we live in has challenged religion to think about some of its basic ideas; and then on the scientific frontier—particularly physics—there has been opposition to the completely materialistic mechanistic way of interpreting this world. So now you get the Paul Davies of this world who are writing about 'The Mind of God' and so on. They are not too clear about what the mind of God is, but at least they are raising questions. The biologists are very different; they are far more mechanistic, and tied to the Newtonian universe.

When I was at Columbia University in the fifties, my chief mentor was Professor Dobzhansky, who was a famous geneticist and evolutionist. At first, he was a bit dubious about my interests. Then he invited me one day to come and have dinner with him. He was Russian by origin. Almost as a confession, he said to me that one of the biggest influences in his life was the Russian Orthodox Church and Dostoevsky. I said, 'Well, you'd be interested in coming to some lectures by Paul Tillich' (who was then at the height of his power—he had just published a book called *Ultimate Concern*). So this distinguished biologist said, 'Well, that's an interesting idea; why should people be concerned about ultimate things?' He then wrote a book called *The Biology of Ultimate Concern*. His colleagues all blamed me for this. They said, 'You've let Charles Birch lead you down the garden path, and there's an abyss at the end of it. You were good before this happened.' It was great fun!

*Were you attacked because of your views?*

No, I wasn't attacked; it was just that they were regarded as a bit odd. There was one guy in particularly who is now one of the brightest biologists in the world. He is a professor at Harvard University, and his name is Richard Lewontin—an agnostic, almost atheist. I said to him once, 'Do you ever question what everything you do adds up to? Is there any purpose beyond just being a lecturer in biology and doing great research?' And he said, 'Charles, when that question crops up in my mind, I go into a room, pull down the blinds, and I try to forget it as quickly as I can.'

*In this period, did you go through stages of doubt?*

All the time. That's the reason I kept on reading and meeting people and being interested. I had tremendous doubts when I left Adelaide to go overseas to Chicago. Maybe it was just a matter of luck that I happened to find myself in the University of Chicago at a time when there was a tremendously powerful group of people in the philosophy and the divinity school. I was in the biology department. Oh, sure, there were doubts.

*Are there doubts now?*

Not generally. I don't want to be dogmatic, but I think I feel fairly confident about the sort of lines that make sense to me.

*Such as?*

Oh, I think I put a great deal of emphasis on the notion of richness of experience, and that the fulfilment of human life is to experience what is potentially possible for life. My idea is that I don't really create that experience, I appropriate it. In other words, there is a source of values beyond myself which I experience and to which I give the name 'God'. God is a persuasive influence, giving goals and purposes at every step. God is persuasive love working in the world.

*Is this God aware of people as individuals?*

Yes. In this notion, God feels every feeling of every creature, every suffering and every joy. And if you ask the question, 'Why doesn't God do something about all the suffering?', I reply that is the most difficult question of the lot. It is the question that fundamentalism cannot answer, except by having the most peculiar distorted theories of atonement. Process thought deals with it along these lines: we are not 100 per cent determined, we have degrees of freedom, and it is a world of chance as well as purpose. If God were to determine the whole thing and remove chance, remove accidents, that would remove the freedom and responsiveness that are the characteristics of human beings. It's not that God has the power to stop the volcano from erupting on the top of a village. God doesn't have that power. It's not in God's nature. God's nature is to suffer with those who suffer in this sort of world.

*As you've become older, have your views changed?*

Compared with other people I know, my views have changed less. There was a framework which I established when I was in my twenties; that framework is still with me, but the details have changed. Oh, one thing that has changed, I've become much more tolerant. I can learn from others who have a very different position.

*What else has changed for you with age?*

Actually, I don't think of growing old, oddly enough. I suppose the main thing that has changed is having less diversity in my life and greater equanimity. I am not put off-track by things that are not really very important. When I was much younger, I couldn't have sat down at a word processor writing something that would go on for a long time. I realised when my mother became old, about eighty, and was living essentially by herself—because my father had died ten years earlier—my concern was that she would become very upset and worried about trivial things that several years before wouldn't have worried her. So one of the things I say to myself is don't be too anxious and worried about the trivial irritations of life that tend to be more aggravating as I get older. I try to control that.

I'll give you a very personal example. One of the things that's always given me a lot of pleasure is to be a resource to people who are in positions that I might have been in when I was much much younger. There's one student in particular that I've been helping in the last few years. He's had a very tragic and difficult life—I dedicated my last book to him—and, because he's had such a tragic environment, I could spend my life worrying about these things. But I try not to. I look at the positive things in terms of the interests I have with him or might help develop in his life. I learn how to be positive instead of negative.

*So do you have a way of dealing with this?*

Not really, no. I try to sit down and think it through, and I suppose what helps me most in these situations is to pull out a book from the book shelves and perhaps read an essay by Paul Tillich, and get back on track again. And then I might say, 'Oh, I'll pass that on, because that might be helpful to him.'

*Do you pray at all?*

Not in the sense of getting down on my knees; no, that's why I don't go to churches any more. I find the performance is not conducive to my having elevated thoughts. The meaning of prayer to me would be to make myself more open and accessible to influences which I think I can appropriate.

I don't meditate. These people who meditate, I can't understand what they do. Lots of them say you've got to get the thoughts out of your head. Well, I've got to get the thoughts into my head, not by sitting alone and looking at the ceiling [laughs], but either by getting into a book or starting to write. I get a lot of thoughts by writing, which is odd. I would never have thought of that ten years ago, when I liked to have everything mapped out beforehand. Now I just sit down at my word processor and, tapping away, I begin to think in ways which wouldn't have happened had I not put them down into the machine. Ten years ago I had to depend upon my terrible handwriting. The word processor makes life so easy.

*You said earlier that you felt now you were more tolerant. What about your tolerance towards institutionalised religion?*

I've become less and less tolerant of that, I'm afraid, but my connection with people is limited in the institutionalised religions. It would be mainly people who are involved in the World Council of Churches, and they are a pretty liberal bunch of people. Their language is still somewhat traditional but their thoughts less so. I find it extremely difficult to be tolerant of the fundamentalist mob in Sydney. I just feel it has a devastatingly bad effect on people. Well, with limitations, because I sometimes ask myself, supposing I'd never been thrown into fundamentalism, would I have ever found a more creative and open sort of religion? Perhaps I wouldn't. Maybe you have to make a mistake before you can find the right thing.

I think this is something which must be very important in parenting. I learned this with students, that you've got to be tolerant of the stupid things that people do and the mistakes they make, realising that it's going to be part of their experience, and you mustn't force them too hard. I remember once saying to a graduate student, 'This is crazy,' and he began to cry, cry, and cry. He said, 'Can't you say something positive?' Students are very upset when they get criticised, but they love their supervisors to say, 'Hey, this is good!' I learned a lesson then which I never forgot.

*You talked about gaining equanimity; is there anything else you've gained with age?*
Yes, I have learned that I don't want to be in a crowd. When I was much younger, I would be more interested in associating with numbers of people. I learned from Paul Ehrlich, who says he never accepts an invitation to a dinner party if there are more than eight people. I think that's a very good maxim. Never go to cocktail parties, because it's just chatter, chatter, chatter. What sort of relationships are going on there? For other people it might be positive and good, but for me it's a total waste of time. I'd be interested in having dinner with a few people—six or seven—but not any more than that, because then you're no longer a group.

I've also learned that it's not important to have a large number of friends, but to have a few that you have a strong rapport with. I don't have a lot of friends. I have a lot of acquaintances, but they don't mean much to me. I'm a monk [chuckles]. I could have lived in a monastery I suppose, whereas earlier on I used to get pretty lonely by myself.

*I wonder why this is?*
Well, I make the distinction between loneliness and solitude. As I grow older, I find that I am much more amenable to times of solitude, perhaps sitting by myself with a word processor, and that's very important. I am alone but I am not alone. I like to be with people if there is some sort of creative interchange going on, but I don't need to be with

people just to be in a crowd. I now experience solitude without loneliness.

*Does this mean that you are now more careful about how you use time, or just that you know what you enjoy?*

I am much more careful. For example, every year for the past thirty or forty years I've been overseas at least once a year, always to a meeting or something. I don't go on holidays. The last couple of years I've said to myself, 'Is this conference really worth going to?' I ask myself that far more carefully and analytically than I would have done even a few years ago, and I partly do that [chuckles] because I find traveling is very tiring. The last two times I went round the world I came back with an awful respiratory infection that I took months to get rid of. That's a high price to pay for going overseas unless you gain a lot, so I no longer have a tremendous urge to travel.

*Are there any aspects of getting old that do worry you?*

There's only one thing, I suppose: I see so many old people whose lives are miserable because of Alzheimer's disease. I have quite a number of friends with Alzheimer's disease—former friends. The first person, who was my real mentor, died twelve months ago, and the last three years of his life were terrible. I'd hate to be in that situation, dependent upon other people, and life's experiences being negative. I have no reason at the moment to feel I am heading in that direction quite, but you never know.

His particular case was that, at the age of eighty, he fell down in the garden and broke his knee. He was shoved into hospital to have the knee set. When they tried to do it with a local anesthetic, he found it very painful and pulled the needle out. So they gave him a general anaesthetic. I learned afterwards that a certain proportion of people from eighty onwards, if they have a general anesthetic, suffer afterwards from a degree of dementia. He never recovered from the operation properly, and he was virtually finished from then onwards. Very sad, because he was intellectually very bright up to that point. He'd had a stroke earlier, which hadn't affected him mentally, but he couldn't anticipate that this catastrophe to his brain would happen following an operation.

*If you'd had early-onset Alzheimer's, and knew you had, would you*

*try to end your life?*
I feel very strongly that absolutes about the sanctity of human life don't help us at all. They help us from avoiding terrible things like Nazi atrocity I suppose, but there has to be some other way of avoiding them. The value of a life for the individual and for God also doesn't have the same value from beginning to end. I don't think a fertilized ovum, one day old, has the same intrinsic value as a mature person. And yet the whole 'Right to Life' movement is based on that hypothesis, which is *ridiculous*. An embryo which doesn't have a nervous system presumably doesn't have much feeling.

Intrinsic values depend upon the capacity for feeling and richness of experience, so intrinsic value in a life would rise like this [indicates], may remain on a plateau for some time, but it doesn't go up for ever. At the onset of Alzheimer's disease it goes down and down—very rapidly and drastically. A person with advanced Alzheimer's is going to be similar to a child that is born with some terrible genetic defect. I respect whatever life is there, but one has to question all the resources that tend to go into these two ends of the spectrum of life to the disadvantage of the rest of society. Hospital expenditure is costly with very elderly people. We have to ask whether that's the best way of using funds.

*Who makes that decision?*
Nobody makes it at the moment, because the hospital accepts anybody who comes in. But it is the big question, and a difficult one. I think the medical profession has learned to make decisions about who should have heart transplants and kidney machines, so that something similar might have to apply in other areas.

*What about if an individual makes a decision that she or he wants to end their life?*
Then I think that's their right. There isn't any absolute moral obligation against that.

*I get back to the question I asked earlier. Do you think you would choose to end your life if you had an illness that was going to be very painful and kill you, or if you had Alzheimer's?*
Provided it didn't cause suffering to other people. But, oh, I don't know; I'd have to judge that at the time. I certainly lay down the rule for myself that I'd want no exceptional medical efforts to keep me alive

if I had something serious wrong with me. I don't think there is any particular value in just eating, breathing, and having my heart beating. That's not life, so I would be against the mainstream of the traditional Christian churches who find euthanasia an anathema. It must be very seriously considered by society and by individuals, and it shouldn't be a crime to commit suicide, nor to help those who want—for good reasons—to end their lives. I know there are all sorts of problems, but we should face them.

*What do you think happens to you after you're dead?*
Ah, well, I don't know. My philosophy requires that something be saved from the whole of the creative process. We know that, according to the second law of thermodynamics, the world is going to be cooked or it's going to freeze. So one way or the other, this world as we know it will finish—a long time in the future, but it's going to finish. What then is the value of the whole creative process? If it all fizzles up into nothing, there is no abiding value. The concept that appeals to me is that a permanent value resides in God. God experiences the creation, God saves what has been created of value in God's own experience. I might say, that seems a bit selfish of God. But God also takes in the suffering as well as the joys.

*Why would God do that if it all fizzles out in the end?*
Because God doesn't fizzle out in the end. God can start a creative process all over again—maybe in another universe, another world, based perhaps not on carbon but on silicon or something.

*Is there a purpose in this world to try and make things better? Are we trying to move towards harmony?*
Absolutely. If the critical thing is the richness of experience in lives, then hopefully people won't be spending their time doing what they are doing in the Balkans at the moment, which seems to be absolutely asinine and insane. People will be spending their time in more creative activities.

*Do you think that will happen?*
There have been great movements for change which have been successful—the anti-slavery movement, anti-child labor movements—but as soon as you solve one problem here, it crops up somewhere else.

So although there are some reasons to be hopeful, I don't think you can guarantee the end is going to be good.

*Did you see Peter Brook's production of the Bhagavad Gita? It gave a sense of the whole cycle of life and death, the richness of life and the re-creation of life, and the fact that, although people kept making the most terrible mistakes, they came up again and again and again—in other words, irrespective of any views on reincarnation it gave a sense of the whole majestic drama of life.*

I think that is one of the most extraordinary things about the whole creative process: that it looks as though the end has come and the dinosaurs are finished, but life starts again from some miserable tiny little creature that has the spark of mammals in it. Life blossoms, time and time again.

*Do you think the essence of Charles Birch will survive?*

No. I think the only contribution I might make in that sense would be to the ongoing life of God. I can't conceive of individual survival. How would you recognise people? Would they be as they were when they were twenty, twenty-one, or when they had Alzheimer's disease? The whole thing doesn't make any sense to me.

What you call 'essence', I'd call 'intrinsic worth'. My friend John Cobb has a mother aged ninety. She's got all her faculties, but keeps on saying to him, 'John I've done all I can; I feel I've made my contribution to the world; I really would be quite happy to lie down and die.' Now, she's still got a lot of intrinsic value in her life; but she thinks that, compared to what it was, she's done her bit. My other friend Charles Hartshorne's wife has Alzheimer's disease, and she doesn't recognise him. He has to regard her as being dead. He gives the impression of not being doubled up with worry about this. 'Don't dwell on it,' he says. He's not going to screw up his own life because his wife has died in a mental way. He says, 'She really died three years ago.' One's value is not the same throughout one's life.

*Isn't that equating the value of a person with the functions they perform?*

No, with the experiences they have. It's not saying that the person is valuable because they do useful things for society—that's a very instrumental way of looking at things, a functional way. A person's value is measured by the richness of the life that they live. That is different. How else would you measure it? Otherwise, you're going to say every bit of life from the fertilised ovum to the last day of Alzheimer's disease is sacred and of infinite value. I don't know how you can say it is of infinite value.

*What have been some of the peaks of your life?*
I get rather surprised when I find the tremendous ups and downs of other people's lives. I am much more on a level. I worked for ten years with Ted Noffs at the Wayside Chapel in Sydney, and I'd wonder how he could have all that enthusiasm and endeavour for something that looked as if it was going to flop anyway. Only one out of ten or twenty of his schemes would be fruitful, but he'd forget about the others. I'm not like that. If I go into a situation, I try to assess it. I say, 'What are my chances of being able to work this out?' Nine times out of ten, I'd say it's not worth my putting effort into it, so I don't.

But then who are the people who change the world? They're the manic people. They're certainly not the people who are in a gulf all the time. I don't think they're the people who are also in the equanimity racket, which is much more comfortable. Certainly, Ted, when he went down, those were terrible moments. I've not experienced that; it seems to be the cost of being manic that you have the great gulf before the next manic period arrives. If it is so, then it's a very big price to pay.

*So is your life reasonably calm?*
Well, it's not all that calm, but I don't have the big highs. Oh, I would have what Abraham Maslow calls peak experiences, but they would have been relatively few. It's not a case of every week that you have a peak experience and then next week you have a gulf, and so on. It's not like that at all. I find that many of my colleagues are very different from that point of view: they get terribly depressed, terribly down, or they get maniacally enthusiastic about something.

*How would you like to be remembered?*
[Laughs] I don't think much about that. I think I'd like to be remembered by the things that have meant most to me, experiences in which I've felt that I've been helpful to other people.

There are some that stand out. The first one was the time in which refugees were coming to Sydney in the forties, boat-loads of them, and

I was involved in something called the World Student Relief Programme. Students were arriving on the boats, former students, they'd been in refugee camps in Europe and prisoner of war camps. We'd arrange to meet them or they would be given information as to how they could get in touch with us. These were situations of absolutely desperate need—students who'd lost their homes, lost friendships, lost everything—and it was very easy to help. Just provide them with friends. Many of them fell by the wayside; some ended up in mental institutions; but many of them came good, found their feet, and struggled against great odds. That was to me a cathartic experience.

One day, my secretary said, 'There is a gold Cadillac at the door; a man wants to see you.' This man said, 'Won't take up much of your time, but ten years ago I came to you from Hungary, and I said I wanted to become a student. The advice you gave me was to go and learn some English, earn some money, and then come back. I did that, and I'm now a millionaire, and if there are any students who are in the position I was in then, I'd like to help them.' That was nice, wasn't it, and really rewarding.

The second time was during the Vietnam War. I'd been in the University of California. I was terribly impressed by the way the staff there had formed a Committee on Conscience and were helping the students who didn't want to be conscripted, and were being sent to jail. The same thing was happening with students in Australia. So I got a group of staff together in Sydney, and we started a Committee on Conscience to provide moral support for students who would otherwise have been very much on their own. This was extremely rewarding. I used to visit kids in Long Bay Jail. I had to go in illegally. I went in with Ted Noffs as his 'assistant chaplain', and gave them messages from their colleagues.

More recently, it would be individuals. After I wrote *On Purpose* I had these curious contacts with young people who were tied up with fundamentalism. One of them who had become extremely sceptical wrote me a letter which said, 'Dear Professor Birch, help!'. He introduced me to others. I got to know quite a lot of these people, and I learned an awful lot myself by association with a group of people who had a point of view which I almost totally rejected, but I hadn't rejected the whole thing. There were values there which were extremely important to them, and I didn't want to disrupt them unduly. I go very carefully when they come to talk to me.

*Will we go on discovering about the nature of life, and how will we go on discovering?*

It's a frontier still. You've got physicists like Paul Davies who admits that every year his mind changes. I think that's true of all of us. The possibilities for the future are enormous, but we've got to discover the language. I have a modicum of reservation, because I never forget Paul Tillich, who was one of the great theologians when I was at Columbia University. Some ten years or so later he said on his death bed, 'Why is it that I am so soon cast on the dust heap of history?' You see, he had been the great influence; every college wanted him to talk. Then, towards the end of his life, other things became important for the Americans. Likewise, there was Reinhold Niebuhr, who was one of the great social thinkers. Nobody now has ever heard of him. People don't read Tillich any more. That's what happens. We're very bad at learning from history. I say this to the World Council of Churches when we have a meeting. I say, we discussed these things in meetings ten years ago; why do we have to do it all over again? Every time, do we have to go back to the beginning again?

*Is a sense of adventure still very much with you?*

Oh, yes, absolutely. I am happy to explore any new insights. I think it's very important to be excited about things that are important. Much better to be excited than to be dull as ditch water.

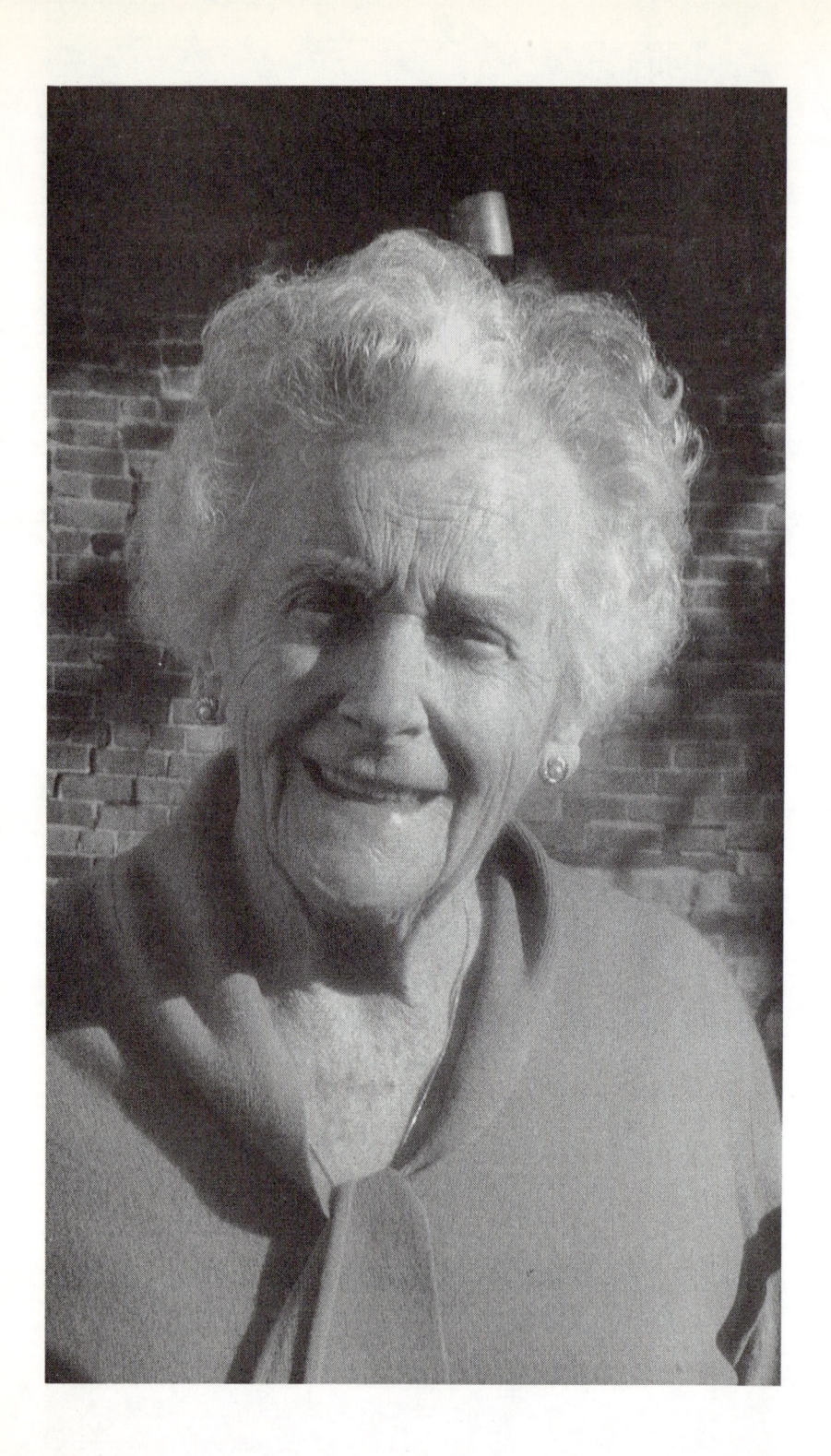

# Nell Forsdyke
*I've had a lot of loving*

Nell Forsdyke was born in Melbourne in August 1910, and spent her childhood in comfort until her father died of self-inflicted gunshot wounds when she was seventeen years old, leaving the family with very little money. She went to teachers' college, and for a long time her teaching helped support her mother, brother, and sister. She married a young banker, Alan, when she was still in her early twenties, had two children, and returned to teaching during the Depression. She started up her own kindergarten, and pioneered the free kindergarten movement in Victoria. Her husband died in 1988, after six years in hospital following a stroke.

For the last three years she has lived in a comfortable residential for elderly people, surrounded by her own possessions, and with regular visits from her family. After her husband's death, she had become increasingly frail, withdrawn, and frightened of living on her own. Every morning, she looks with joy at one of her paintings of the Australian landscape because it allows her to 'walk through the painting' and out again into her beloved bush. She talks now in a small, hesitant voice; but, although much of her short-term memory has gone, she has dignity and clarity about the important things in her life.

I had a very happy childhood. We lived at Fairfield. We had a lovely garden. It went right down to the river. It was the second marriage for my father and my mother, and it was a very happy marriage. I was their first child. And the night my father died, my older sister told me she wasn't my sister. It was a big shock: I lost a father and a sister. Can you understand that? But then we grew up to be wonderful friends. She had very good taste. I felt I was a draught horse, but she just seemed to be gifted in interior decorating and arranging furniture. One day she came and, while I was out in the kitchen getting lunch, she just moved everything around my sitting room. I had an aunt there who was quite shocked. She said, 'You can't do that in Nell's house, Margery.' However, she did, and the room looked miles better.

*What were some of your earliest memories?*

Mother had a Seventh Day Adventist step-father, and of course they didn't eat meat. So she had a wonderful education, unusually detailed in food values for that time. I think we were very well children.

*So you didn't eat meat as a child?*

Oh, yes. Father wasn't a Seventh Day Adventist. But mother had learned from her mother, the Seventh Day Adventist, the value of raw food—salads and vegetables and all those sorts of things.

*Were your mother and father strict?*

They were firm. There was no nonsense, but I had a very happy life even though they should have told me things sooner. The night my father died, my sister turned to me and said he wasn't my father. I always made up my mind that if I had children, if there was any family history I'd tell them.

*What sort of games did you play?*

We had an Edison Bell record machine, and it had marches on it, and we'd march around the sitting room and in and out the doors. We loved that. When we went to our next house at Rye there were sandcastles, and I loved my Rye days. We went down to Rye in the influenza epidemic and we stayed on. I think it was those times at Rye that made me Australian. I loved the bush. I knew where the mushrooms grew, and the orchids. I had an older sister and a younger sister and a brother. Perhaps it was a bit lonely, our childhood. Mother was very particular about with whom we played, but I always felt very secure and very happy.

*What did your father do?*
He lived on his money.

*How had he made his money?*
It was left to him, and that was wrong. Never do that. My father was a clever man. He loved music.

*So did you have a lot of music in the home?*
A lot of singing, yes. Mother sang soprano: 'Come into the garden, Maude' was one of them. I think it was very Victorian sort of music. We used to waltz around the piano and the gramophone.

*Do you remember the clothes you wore?*
I remember the very first casual clothes we had. I had a very modern aunt, and she said to mother, 'Elsie, you're hopelessly old fashioned. Your children should have play clothes,' because we were still in starched clothes. I remember we had blue lustre frocks; I can still feel them scratching. They were embroidered with a red thread round the neck, and we had red belts. Mother thought they were dreadful clothes but that was what the well-dressed children, according to my aunt, were wearing. Oh yes, and I can remember the starching that went on, and black patent leather shoes. Your best clothes were only worn on Sundays and on family events. Mother had good help—old Ellen. Mother had advertised for help, and when the relatives brought Ellen down she was so downtrodden that mother's heart went out to her. I loved old Ellen. She'd let me spend Saturday afternoons doing her long hair, and yet she often referred to me as 'that Nell'.

*So were you a mischievous little girl?*
I think I was very active. I loved flowers. Father would plant out a bed of flowers, or let me plant them, and I'd pull them up every day to see if the roots were forming. I was very secure, and we had freedom within clearly defined limits. We went to bed when we were told. They sent me to school when I was four and a half, and I loved it. I found the mystery of … of how words were made. See, I learned sounds—'aih',

'eih', 'ih', 'oh', 'ah'. I went to a little school called Alexander College in Westgarth, and Mr Farr was very strict. He'd thump you on the back. He thumped my young brother, whom I loved dearly, and I said, 'Mr Farr, if you thump my brother again, my mother will take us all away from this school.' He never thumped again. I won a scholarship to Melbourne High, the J Kitchen and Sons scholarship. I could write essays at the drop of a hat. I loved Melbourne High.

*What did you look like when you were a young girl?*
I was always inclined to be plump. Mother took great pride in our complexion, our skin, and our hair. I'm sure we were the cleanest children that ever existed. When I was very young my hair was quite red—golden, mother told me it was. But that rubbed off, and then I had ordinary brown hair, but it always behaved itself for me. I haven't thought of the colour of my hair for years.

*How old were you when you first became interested in boys?*
See, I had a brother, and I had cousins, and boys would seem to be quite a natural part of my life, do you understand? I used to think, 'Oh, I don't s'pose I'll ... you know, I'm a bit fat.' When I met my husband I knew he was going to be special. I used to think to myself, 'If I haven't met someone by the time I'm twenty-one then I'll begin to get worried.' But I met him just before my twenty-first birthday. He was a quiet man, but I really think he was the kindest, gentlest person I've ever known. I think everybody loved Alan. He was absolutely trustworthy, and a banker, and very secure.

*You said that when you saw him you knew he was the one. Can you describe that feeling?*
I was just beginning to sing, and I was learning from Dorothy Humphries, who was one of our best sopranos. She always sang solo in the Messiah performance at Christmas time in the Town Hall. She was very pleased apparently with the progress I was making, and then I was asked to sing at Footscray for the young Presbyterians. This was my first appearance. My sister had just been married, and I had a very pretty bridesmaid's frock. They rang me up and said, 'Wear evening dress.' So I put on my very soft green chantilly lace frock, and when I got there it was in the Town Hall. It was packed, and suddenly there was a whirlwind—violin, you know—and on the tick of eight Alan

walked onto the platform to open the concert, and I thought, 'He can play!' That's my first impression.

The Mayor of Footscray asked us to repeat the concert for the unemployed. So Alan came up and sat next to me, and he said, 'Miss Hassell?' And I said, 'Yes.' And he said, 'You're from Fairfield.' And I said, 'Yes.' And he said, 'Do you know the Thompsons in Fairfield, Sylvia and Eric?' 'Oh,' I said, 'indeed I do, very well.' He couldn't have offered a better reference. They both went to my church. They were very nice, brother and sister, and that was Alan's cousins. So that's really the first time I had a good look at him. He was such a gentle man.

*And when did he ask you out?*

He asked me to go to Faust, and my sister loaned me this lovely blue velvet evening coat. And then he began to ask me out regularly. I invited him to my twenty-first birthday party. He was very quiet then, very well groomed, quietly spoken but absolutely, completely, and utterly reliable.

*Was he older than you?*

About four years, I think.

*And how long did you spend going out with each other before you became married?*

It was about eighteen months, I think. I'd had a lot of sadness: my father had died, so father didn't ever know Alan, but mother loved him. He was a very quiet man. I've got his photo somewhere. And steadfast.

*Did you go to university?*

No, but I went to teachers' college. I could have gone on to university, but it was just impossible. My father died that year, and no income, no money, and … I think he took his own life. See, he'd been brought up as a rich man's son, never given any training. 'My sons will never have to work for a living!'—that's what our grandpa said, which was so wrong. And I think he began to be so ill; oh, he was in such pain with a gall bladder. I begged him to go to the doctor, but I don't think he could afford it, I think there was no money. You know the wonderful thing was the way the family, the Hislop family, stuck together. And how my aunt said, 'Nell, if only he'd told us.' My aunt took over the mortgage—the house was mortgaged! We didn't know that!

*When you were a young woman, in the thirties there was the great economic depression. Were you conscious of people living in poverty?*
But Alan was a bank manager, a banker, and he was such a good manager and I, if I may say, I could manage, too.

*Was your marriage a happy one?*
Very, I was so secure.

*Did you enjoy being a mother?*
Loved it. Marg, look, she was everything a daughter could be. She was a pretty girl. She missed red hair by the skin of her teeth, and she was very bright.

*Did you have help with the children?*
Oh yes, we had—oh, I forget her name—but she used to come and do the washing and the ironing, and I had the house cleaned on Fridays.

*Were there any dark periods in your marriage, or in your life?*
I always felt that once I met Alan my life was secure, straightforward, and happy. Look, he was the most selfless man—very generous, generous to a fault. When I went back to teaching, the Thompsons were shocked. They said things like, 'Of course, it's a reflection on Alan that you can't manage to live on his salary!' And then, by the greatest stroke of good luck, in my teaching I got a very backward little boy, and I thought to myself, 'You're not backward at all; you're just withdrawn.' I set to work on this child, worked really hard. I loved teaching, and they were short of teachers, so I went back to teaching after Alan died. No, I think I went back before he died. Yes, oh yes, I went to Corowa, the girl's grammar school, and we had a revolution in religious teaching.

*When did Alan die? Long ago?*
It feels like a million years.

*Has it been hard since?*
It's extraordinary. I think I must just have closed the book and said that was a good life, now get on ... I ... I'm trying to be completely

honest with you. And of course I've had such support from my family.

*And tell me what it feels like now. Do you feel old? Or do you feel just the same inside?*

I think I feel just the same and yet … I'm trying … it's so hard to be completely honest with you … I'm … I feel very secure and comfortable and I have no anxieties; and Marg and Tom and Don and Cathy, my family, I think, 'Well, they're happy, they're good citizens'—which used to be my favourite phrase. I used to say often to my children, 'Learn to be a good citizen.' I don't think I've felt alone.

*Do you feel frightened about losing your memory?*

Yes. And then the other half of me says, 'So what?' See, I have lived longer than any member of my family. No one else has had an eightieth birthday. I think I accept it. I'm very comfy, looked after, no anxieties.

*Can you tell me what it's like when you can't remember things?*

It never worries me. I think I say, 'Oh well, I'm getting old.' I hope this doesn't sound like Bible banging, but I really have faith. It's an everyday thing: I'm God's child. I think I'm speaking truthfully when I say I feel secure.

*Marg has said that sometimes you think that maybe people are trying to hurt you, and you get worried and frightened.*

Well, I can't remember that. But I'd like her to tell me. Of course, if it's important for me to remember things, I have my little … see, I write it down [rustle of paper]. Apparently I haven't had anything important to remember. But I do. If it's very important that I remember I write it down. See … what I've written here on Wednesday, the fourteenth of April—that was at twenty-eight past eight in the evening:

> Marg came this evening, absolutely ladened with lovely fresh, clean, ironed and mended winter clothing. She hung it up and took some of the summer clothes I probably don't need. Then Marg left and I spent the rest of the evening in the sitting room. I had tea at Hedley Sutton. Margie left and after tea I went to television with Dorothy and Doreen Homes. I came back to my room but there is no money at all. No money at all. The coin purse has gone and with it any small change I had. The black patent leather bag was completely empty. I think a couple of dollars. I took …

Now that was in April, 1993. And I have absolutely no recollection of it.

*Did you feel then that somebody was stealing your purse?*
Yes, I must—because I never leave my purse in the room. I keep it with me all the time. I put it under my pillow at night, and I haven't lost anything more. Anything very special of mine—that's right, I had a lot of lovely crystal and stuff—I begged Marg to take it. And I think I ... sometimes I think I might make it up; but I'm not too sure about that.

*You think somebody might be stealing things around the place?*
Yes ... I don't know ...

*And what about your physical health? How is that?*
I feel very well. I sleep all night, and I eat well, and I try not to eat too well. I weigh on the scales, regularly. I walk—I can't bear strolling. And ...I feel I'm well. But again, you see, you don't know whether you're ... oh, I must be. I don't know. You really can't trust yourself, I think. That's where Marg's so good.

*You can't trust yourself?*
To remember. You see, I don't think I've made any errors in talking to you. I hope I haven't. But I do use the old pencil and paper quite a lot, and I find that's a help. I don't think I'm frightened. I think I'm ... well, I'm ageing, and that's it.

*Are you frightened of dying?*
No, no. I've loved my church and the church teaching, and I'd hate to be ill for a long time but it's out of your hands. I've lived longer than any of my relatives.

*You sound quite pleased about that!*
I marvel at it. I think, you know, why me? And I'm ... peaceful here, and I feel I'm not a nuisance. Oh, I didn't want to be a nuisance. I wouldn't. I ... I don't ... I would not want Marg to do one thing less than she's doing, because I didn't want her to feel she's got to see me or do this or do that. That's fair enough, isn't it? And because ... I had such ... the Thompsons were so very difficult ... and yet they gave me lovely gifts. He was a jeweller, Alan's father, and this is my engagement

ring. But anything else I don't keep here, only the things I can wear.

*How do you think you'd like to be remembered?*

Now this is being Goddy, but I ... I think Christian teaching of sharing and loving and giving has been very important to me, and yet you do meet awful wowsers. I hope I'm not a wowser. But nevertheless the fact that God is love has been a very important part of my life, and wherever there's been real love and real affection there's God. I think that's as honest an expression I can make. Because, you see, I've had a very loving husband, I've got Marg and Don and Tom and Cathy. I feel I've had a lot of loving.

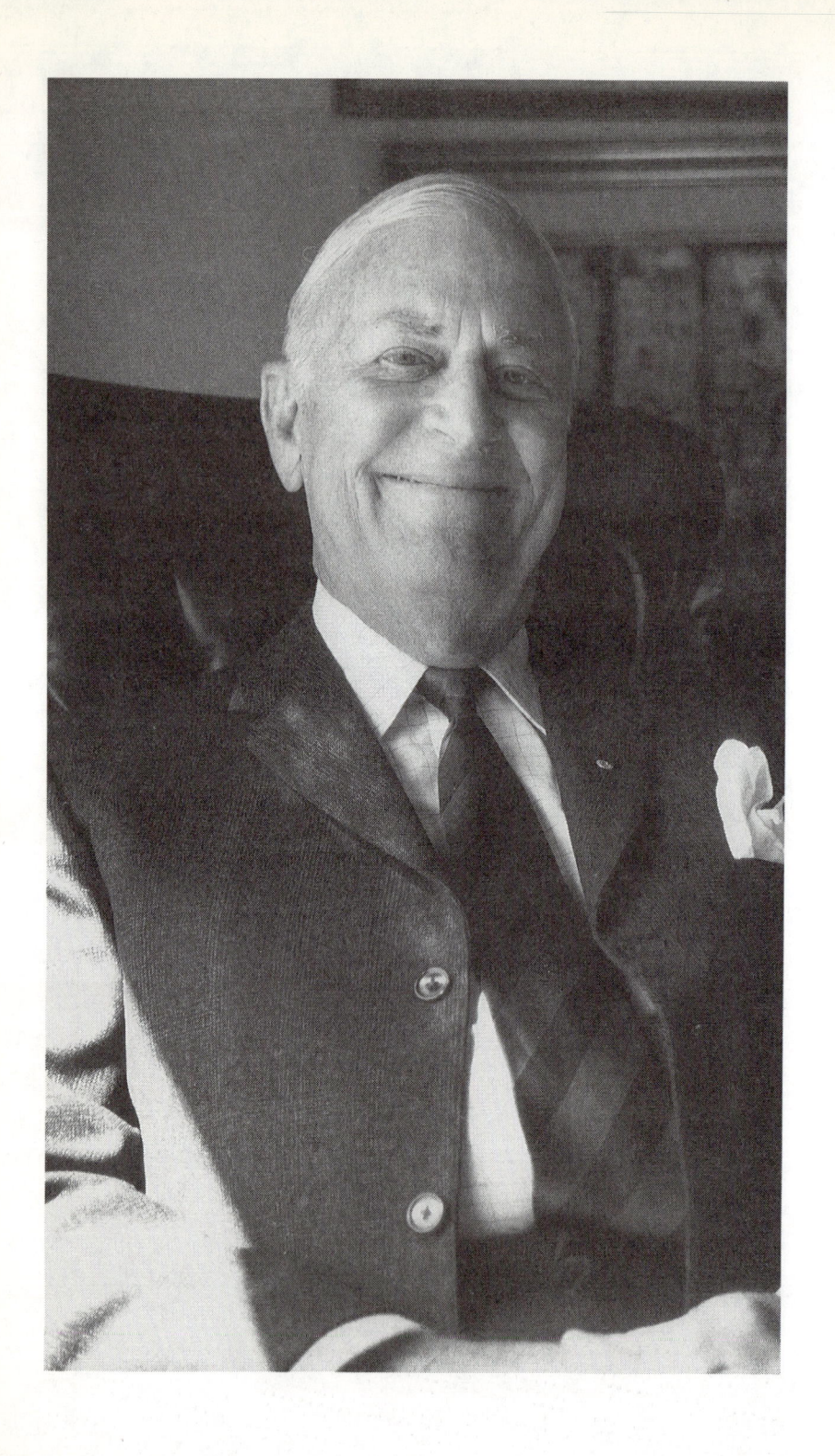

# Leycester Meares
*Never let anything go that you believe in*

Leycester Devenish Meares, AC, CMG, QC, had a distinguished legal career. He served on numbers of government councils, tribunals, and boards, including being chairman of the New South Wales Law Reform Commission, chairman of the National Advisory Council for the Handicapped, chairman of the Foundation of Australian Resources, and chairman of the Australian Vietnam War Veterans Trust. From 1969 to 1979, he was a judge of the Supreme Court of New South Wales.

When I first met him, he was chairman of the National Advisory Council for the Handicapped, and his optimism and energy were impossible to ignore. By the time I conducted this interview, he was in his eighties and, not well, spent much of his time at home in his Kirribilli apartment overlooking the harbour. But he still had the same convincing enthusiasms and concerns.

Leycester Meares was born in Sydney in January 1909. He died in August 1990, at the age of eighty-five, as this book was being prepared for press.

I am *infinitely* wiser than I was fifty years ago. I can suffer things. I understand how people tick much more. I don't hate anybody any longer, because I think I can understand why they're doing certain things. That's not because of ability. It's simply as the result of experience. To me, life with increasing age has been much, much easier.

*Does this mean it's been much better for you?*

Yes. I've done more with my life in the last thirty or forty years, I think, than before. I'm very fortunate, because 'me' is unimportant. I don't have any worries about 'me' whatsoever; and, although nobody will ever believe me, I've never had any ambitions. Things just happen. A door opens: then it closes and another door opens. I have felt about my life that I have about as much control of it as a match thrown into a whirlpool.

*Did you ever try to control it?*

Only when I was young and stupid, up to the age of twenty-three, twenty-four; but after, never. I don't believe in destiny. Things just happen in one's life. You have an opportunity and you pick it up, and you do what you can with it. And that is what life has been for me. As one thing finishes, another opportunity arises. That is why life has been full of challenges, excitements, disappointments, and sometimes results.

*When you were a child, did you have old people around who were significant in your life?*

Never. I never really knew my father, who was a marvellous person and very successful. I was infinitely closer to my mother, and I think she loved me rather much. But then I had four brothers—two older, two younger—and I was influenced by them I think in pre-adolescence and, later, in family life.

*What did your father do?*

He was general manager of a huge co-operative, The Producers Co-operative Distributing Society Ltd; he was president of the Chamber of Commerce; he was this, this, and this. He lived and died for the principle of co-operative marketing, but that principle has been one that has not succeeded. Father succeeded only because of father. One thing I've learned in the last half century, as a result of being on dozens of charitable committees, is that for any committee to be successful it must have a chairman with a lot of drive, and/or an executive officer with the same ability. Otherwise it will just do nothing.

*What made you go into the law?*

I had a great friend—it was a David and Jonathan relationship—we simply lived in each other's pockets since we were three. Everybody used to laugh at us because we were never apart. His father was a barrister, and perhaps I was influenced by that fact, but I was always an immensely argumentative, wretched creature, and everybody knew that I had to be a lawyer. I never had any other ambition; never.

*So for you the law was a good choice?*

The only choice.

*You've talked several times already about zip and energy and vitality. Is this something you've always had a good measure of?*

Yes, I believe it's one of the few qualities I possess. I'm not an exceptionally intelligent person, and the talents that I've had I've really had to make the most of. I've lacked the advantages of people with first-class brains, and I suppose that has meant in my life much more work than some others. But the law has always been my first love.

*Is vitality important to success, do you think?*

In my case, people tell me I have always been an impatient person who never keeps still. This is a quality that one's friends complain of, that I don't know much about. But my life, its incentives and initiatives and dreams, and the ambition to see that those dreams come true, is not just physical energy. It is something that is part of me For instance, the Child Accident Prevention Foundation is a charity that is now twelve years old. Margaret Guilfoyle, the Minister for Social Security, asked me to grab it and do something about it. I suppose for about six years I would go down to Melbourne to meetings, and when I would come back I would think, 'Oh, I'm just wasting my time.' But I just kept on, and the Foundation is a dream that's come true. I still have things happening in projects that I had a lot to do with many years ago. Success has often been a result of dripping water on stone; it's terribly exciting when one hears of a tremendous result after years and years.

*So is persistence important as well?*

Oh, hell yes; absolutely vital. Never let anything go that you believe in. Without that I would never have got anywhere. Despite disappointment after disappointment, failure after failure, lack of achieving what you want to achieve, you never want to give in. That's the only way I've achieved results.

*Did any of this discipline and self-service come from your family, from your mother or your father?*

Well, father had it to a great degree, but I never acquired it until after the war. Until I was thirty, thirty-five, I was immensely self-centred in early days. And then the war came, and that was quite an experience. I think in the war I learned the importance of loving: that it was only by truly caring for my men that one could earn their loyalty. I think that was when I was imbued by a sense of service to others. I can't teach people this; but happiness, as you would know, is as elusive as a sunbeam. To hold it is like holding quicksilver. But my happiness—and it has been substantial—has come from service to others, certainly not from worrying about myself. That's been a terrific blessing I've had, not having to worry about myself. I don't ever look in the mirror.

*But have you never—literally—looked in the mirror and thought, 'Oh God, I'm getting old'?*

Well I've got old, but I don't look back. In my whole life, I've never looked back. and that's just how one is made. I've always looked forward. Now I'm looking forward I think to the end of a life, but without any fear. I do not fear death, but I fear dying if that proved difficult.

*In terms of physical pain or indignity?*

Both, but mainly in terms of indignity. That's what I fear. You know, we used to pray in the litany to be spared from sudden death. It was just one of those ridiculous beliefs we had that nobody presently shares.

*Do you believe that the taking of one's own life should be allowed?*

Yes, I don't have any doubt about it. But it's very difficult to legislate for. I think some countries are experiencing that difficulty. For instance, a paraplegic or a quadriplegic, in the first six or nine months of their paraplegia or quadriplegia, should not be allowed to elect to die, a time in which so many of them feel so dreadful; but as time goes on they adjust. But for the old, yes. As chairman of the federal government's

National Advisory Council for the Handicapped, for some ten years or so, I suppose I visited dozens and dozens of nursing homes. Most of those with Alzheimer's disease or senile dementia are not in any true sense living—they are merely existing—but the difficulty with them is who should be allowed to decide the question.

*Do you believe that our attitudes towards people who are old are getting better?*

No question of that, as are our attitudes towards people with handicaps or, as they say now, disabilities. The attitude of Australians in relation to the disabled has changed dramatically in the last twenty-five years, to my knowledge. I believe that, as far as the aged are concerned, we are adopting perhaps slightly more the Asian philosophy towards them: that they must be cared for and looked after in their homes. Institutional care, wherever practical, should cease to exist.

*You were very firm about that. Nobody's going to get you into an institution! When we talk about 'cared for' and 'looked after', that also has its hazards, because you can look after somebody and take away their independence, which you must have seen in many of the homes you've visited.*

I think with the abandonment of institutional care, wherever practicable, people with disabilities are having more say in their living, but even in group homes they still often will lack independence. I don't think that the aged, generally, will ever be completely independent. I think that, as the years run down, one's independence decreases; but nobody interferes with me yet, thank goodness.

*Yes, but sometimes it's in such small things. I can remember a discussion centred around whether somebody should be forced to have jelly with their custard or not, which is symptomatic of an attitude where often quite small choices are taken away from old people, and they are treated as if they're babies.*

I don't think there's any doubt about that. The older they get, the less competent—physically or mentally—and the greater the tendency of those who love them to control them. A lot of old people, as a result of their abilities decreasing, accept this; but the very independent have to suffer. Speaking for oneself, I've always fought bitterly against it, so far successfully.

*Has anyone ever tried to tell you what to do or to treat you with condescension?*

No, no. I'm not made that way, and I think one's friends appreciate it. My secretaries have been magical. My present secretary, she knows more about me than I do; she does so much for me, and I wonder how I would get on without her. She treats me not with condescension, but as one who still has decisions to make.

*Do you think that in Australia we have a cult of youth and this makes it harder for old people?*

Anne, dear, I don't see enough of youth to form a view about that. I have young friends, and they stimulate me, and I think I can get farther with them than some others. I seem to have a natural empathy with them. But from what I see of them, I think that the present younger generation is better than my generation.

*Do you have any particular religious beliefs?*

No. My mother used to speak of 'the parish'. She was an English woman, and we were dragged to church until we had left home. But I cannot believe—although I have tried—in a personal God. I have given it a lot of thought. I suppose most people have. But the interesting part about belief that I have difficulty with is that, in every country, every race believes in some superior being. That's the only argument to me in favour of some superiority, some force; but I remain agnostic.

*Do you ever ponder about the meaning of life?*

No. It's about nothing. We are a form of life which is superior to other forms of life. But, looking at the universe, I don't really think in many ways we're more important than an ant. We live and we die. We have greater personalities, greater intellect, greater abilities than all other forms of life. But we're simply a form, although a superior form, of life. The human species has been defined as an environmental abnormality. Whether this be true or not, we are the world's greatest polluters. I don't think that life *per se* has any meaning, but I believe that it is well-lived by observing the ten commandments.

*Yet those are biblical injunctions.*

Whether they be biblical or otherwise, those ten commandments are wise commandments, no matter who thought of them. I don't relate to them spiritually; but I think if we all lived by the commandments, life would be much better for us all.

*But then why is it important to live well? Why do we try to be 'good'?*

The fact that we have to live with other people, whether in a dormitory when one is young, or in a profession or trade when one gets older, you simply must listen to the other person's point of view and accept their importance. I think that's the art of living, to appreciate the other fellow's point of view and to understand him. With age, usually that becomes easier.

*You referred earlier to the fact that you no longer hated. Did you, as a young man?*

Yes, I hated; not abnormally, but I did hate. Those days are quite gone. I don't any longer hate, and it makes life so much easier. I don't know whether this is something that happens as a result of age, but it certainly happened with me.

*You showed me a painting in your apartment of a young man who you said was 'a bad egg'; he had a glowering expression. When you get young people who appear to be 'bad eggs', do you believe that can be changed with love?*

Yes, I do ... but assessing what is right or wrong, I find very difficult. What was right twenty years ago is wrong today, and vice versa. There are plenty of examples of sexual mores to prove that. I believe that there is nothing more important than a happy home life, at least until the age of adolescence. The very great proportion of those so advantaged live with sound principles and are, so to speak, insulated against many of the pitfalls of life. A truly happy home life and the teaching of proper principles simply clads a person with a protection against going wrong. I believe that with many criminals it's not their fault but the gamut of their environment and upbringing. There is, I think a tremendous amount of truth in the saying, 'There but for the grace of God go I.'

*Did this make it difficult for you as a judge?*

Sometimes. I think that many of the criminals knew how one was feeling, and one's sympathies for them, but there was a job to be done. Sentencing is a terribly difficult task. It has to be done, but it has to be done to a large percentage of the criminal population who are simply the victims of circumstances.

*Can the law ever rehabilitate people?*

I've always wanted to be a student of penology, but I've never had the time. I believe that our present system of punishment, and our present jails system and keeping people contained, is a system in which rehabilitation is very difficult. I don't think it's something we have succeeded in. I think that what you want in a jail is loving, and I don't think under our system over the last fifty years there's been much loving; certainly not on the part of the warders.

*And the legal profession itself; would you like to see changes there?*

Our administration of justice in the courts, in my view, is a laugh. It is chaotic and ridiculous. I think that if we had a metaphorical man from Mars coming down here, and we had to tell him that if a person were committed for trial and granted bail, that he had to wait for three years to be tried; or that if bail was refused and a man was incarcerated, that he had to wait for a year to be tried; or that if he had an accident and he thought it was somebody else's fault, that he had to wait from two to four years to get a judgment; or if he knew that the cost of litigation rendered it beyond the reach of anybody but the very rich and those with legal aid, I think the man from Mars would scream with demoniacal laughter. In other words, our system has hopelessly failed.

*Does that depress you?*

Yes. Anthony Sampson once said of the legal profession that they were entrapped in their own conservatism. That has been my own experience.

*You've talked a lot about love and loving; is this something you've had in you own life?*

Yes. I have a wide circle of friends, of all social strata, and I believe that we love each other. Loving comes from extending oneself in the interest of others, caring. If you have a relationship with a person and you really worry about that person, that's half the battle. Without true caring and concern, friendships are not really valuable.

*Do you ever wish you'd had children?*

Yes. And the older you get, without becoming in any way paedophilic, you love little children. They are Australia's greatest asset. They need all our attention and help and love and care.

*If you measure your life in terms of outstanding peaks, what have they been?*
Well, I think of being made a companion in the Order of Australia; I think of being made a lieutenant-colonel in the army; of being the first president of the Australian Bar Association; being made a Queen's Counsel, and then a judge; and being made an Anzac of the Year. I suppose these are peaks. But, oh dear, they've never really made me feel important or thrilled me for more than a matter of weeks—they really haven't.

*And troughs?*
I can't really remember any dreadful troughs. There have always been silver linings. I've never struck a trough that was so deep that I could not climb out.

*What other things give you delight now?*
One's friends, and an increasing interest in art.

*Are there things that you still want to do?*
No, no. I've had a very fortunate life, so there's nothing that I really regret, and nothing that I would really wish to do. I don't suffer a great deal of frustration. If sometimes I do look back in wakeless hours of night, I can only then truly recall all of my dreadful mistakes. But I don't wish to try again.

*How would you like to be remembered?*
This is a question I find of little interest. If I have to answer it, I suppose I'd like to be remembered not as a successful lawyer, nor as a person who'd achieved this or that, but as a person who had qualities as a human being.

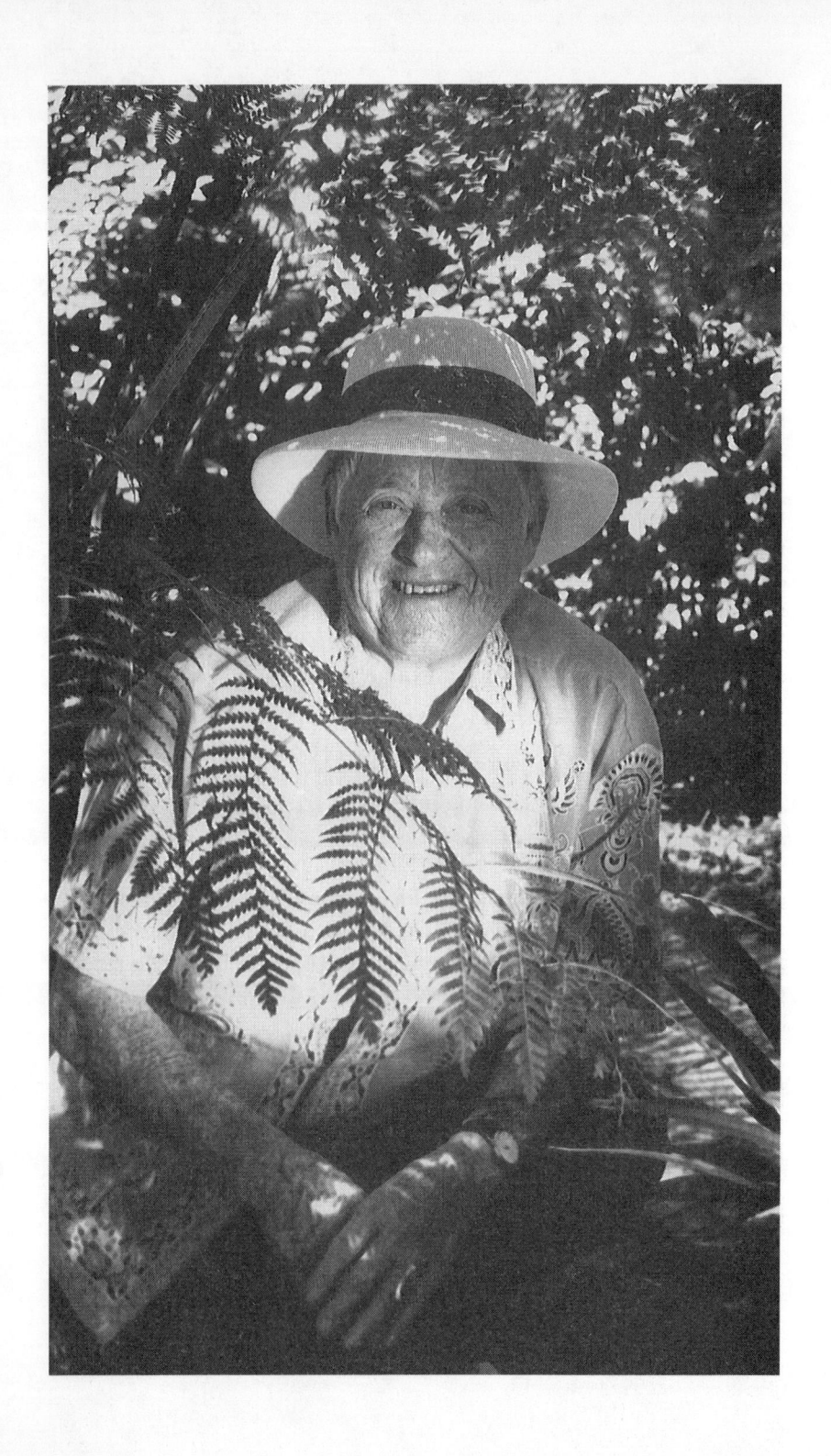

# Margaret Jones
*Woman warrior*

Margaret Jones, arts student at Macquarie University, will be seventy-five when she gets her first degree. Before she went to university, she worked for many years as a legal secretary, 'the wise old workhorse that launched the careers of a dozen articled clerks.'

Margaret Jones doubly deserves the title 'Woman Warrior'. She is a warrior for confronting her fear of formal education and a sense of powerlessness; and she is also a warrior for being a public lesbian at a cost to her sense of social belonging.

She was born into the parish of the Church of St Mary Immaculate at Manly, New South Wales in April 1927 and, in her own words, was 'baptised there, christened, confirmed, confessed, received absolution, re-sinned, re-absolved, observed the sacraments there,' and heard the reading of her bans of marriage to a Hungarian country boy from Pecs.

Then she left—first of all the Catholic church, and then the country boy. She talks about society's alienation of her as a new Australian bride and society's further alienation of her as a 'dirty dyke'. She is angry about the failure to educate women of the 1920s, and considers it has restricted and limited her life. She lives in an inner-city suburb of Sydney, and enjoys spending time in her garden.

I can remember my old aunts and a grandmother. When we'd greet them, I was always a little reluctant to be embraced by them. I looked at them as quite old and crinkly, and not very cuddly and embraceable. I liked them all right; it was just because they were old. My parents were ordinary parent age. I didn't see them as old, old, old.

*That sense of old people being somehow distasteful; do you think that's the same now?*
More so now. Because this is the age of the young. All the images, advertising and the media, entertainment, are around the young and their interests. So they tend to think we're even older than we are.

*I remember my younger son, when he was about four, saying to me, 'Are you very old?' I said, 'No, not yet,' and he said, 'That's okay. I didn't think you were 'cause you smell quite fresh to me.'*
That's very perceptive at age four.

*Can you remember a time when you first became conscious that you were getting older?*
Yes, I can: only ten years ago, which would be about fifty-five. I don't think I saw it physically. I've been always pretty fit and healthy, and I move quickly. I think I just looked older, and started to grey, and then began to get different treatment from people—disregarding and talking to me in another way. So ten years ago I started to age.

*How did that affect you?*
Oh, I was good and mad [laughter]. I didn't think I was *that* old that I had to be deferred to or patronised. So I have a lot of anger about that, anger that I haven't dealt with. My anger doesn't abate; it only gets worse as the older I get the treatment of me is worse.

*Can you remember any examples?*
Yes, a great many. In my business I go into a lot of offices, and I announce myself: 'Hello, I'm Margaret Jones.' And they instantly say, 'Yes, Mrs Jones.' I gently try to ask how could they *presume* that I was married, and could they use the term "Ms". And a few of them— probably because of me getting vexed—have said, 'Oh yes, I thought you were a "Mrs," and that you'd be angry if I called you a "Miss" '—

suggesting that a Miss has missed out, missed out on matrimony. Now that's my first memory of being called a "Mrs"' when I hadn't before, when I had red hair not grey.

*Do you think older people get a worse deal now than they did in the past?*

I believe we do. I'm now locked into a youthful world because I'm a mature-age student at a university in Sydney. The great proportion of first-year students are straight out of school, seventeen and eighteen, and I'm the only person in the lecture rooms and the tutorials that's old and grey. I'm surrounded by youth. I see their interests are not mine, and I'm no part of them. They don't even engage me in conversation. I'm totally invisible.

*So they don't react with you?*

No, no, no.

*Do you make any attempt to react with them?*

I do. At first, I was full of good cheer, and I'd bustle in, 'Hello hello,' and smile, and they'd just grudgingly nod or look. I kept forcing myself to do that, and then I quit. So I know it can now be said that, because I don't say 'hello' to them, I can't expect them to 'hello' back. They 'hello' to each other; they have the ability. I've seen them open their mouth and say, 'Hi.' So perhaps if I get some more courage, I might try talking to them again and seeing if they *will* respond. Even if they do, when I get them to talk, they won't know what to say to this old, old woman. What could they say that she could know about? How could she relate to them? So, for all of those reasons, they wouldn't want to engage with me. I've got nothing to give them—so they think.

*What have you got to give them?*

I could talk about my interests in my life, and I could hear about their's. And sure as hell they could give me some answers to the bloody essays. They don't, and I miss that network. I see them chattering to each other, and swapping notes, and helping each other, and reading together—and not one of them offers me any help. So if I were … nicer, if that's the word, then they might give me some help. But that's what I think I could give to them, too: perhaps to tell them that I'm not as *boring* as they think I am, that I've lived quite an exciting and different life.

*This must be quite alienating.*

Oh, it is. The whole university experience is, the youth of them, the fact that I'm ignored by them. And the lecturers—look, I shouldn't expect them to take any more notice of me than the younger ones, but even they don't seem to have an awareness that I might need a bit more help or encouragement because of my age, and that it takes me longer to understand what's required of my readings. So between the lot of them, the lecturers and the kids, it's tough going being a mature-age student.

*Why did you make this decision?*

To be a mature-age student? Well, as I'd come to the end of any meaningful paid work that I could do, I became very isolated and frustrated and in depression, with nothing to do and endless, endless time to fill in. I did it for something to do, which I now see isn't enough reason. There's no motivation. When things get tough, I don't know how to impel myself to study harder —because I've got no reason to be a BA.

*But what about the actual process of learning? Are you getting something out of that?*

Yeah, well, I've sure discovered my ignorance. But it's very hard; it has no relevance to me. What I'm learning is introduction to behavioural science, and anthropology, sociology, and words and concepts and stuff I've never even heard of. It's like I'm starting from the beginning of primary Catholic school in the 1930s. I don't even have any sense of the concept of what it is; whereas the kids do, they were doing that all that last year in HSC. Even words I don't understand—I have to scurry off and find what a word means, and then I've missed the context of it because I'm worrying about this word. I find it very difficult, not having had any education for fifty years, to suddenly be dumped into it all.

*Will you continue?*

Oh, I must. Because otherwise I'm back to where I was, which was depression. I'm doing only two subjects a year, so there goes ten years before I'm finished. You know, I have to have sixty points; if I'm getting six a year I'll be there till … 2010 [laughter].

*Going back to that period when you were in your fifties and you suddenly realised you were getting older, your hair was going ... white, how did it affect you, that physical change?*

Yeah, well, because I felt so energetic and healthy, the change was an external nuisance, but I didn't feel it within myself. I felt quite happy and cheerful and content with my life.

*And now?*

Now I feel bad about myself, so I have to feel bad about my age.

*But physically are you still fit and healthy?*

Oh, yes. I believe that I am. I move quickly, and I do walking and exercise and aquarobics, so I think that I'm quite healthy .

*Do you mind that sense of growing physical deterioration?*

Yes. I don't like looking at my skin and the loose folds of it, and my fallen breasts and my sunken pieces. I don't like the look of me.

*So how do you try and cope with that?*

Well, I can't alter it; it's there. I just wear long sleeves, which hides it. But then I'm angry at myself for doing that. I don't need to hide it, and people know it, surely. People know it's there because they look at my face, and see my age, and must imagine I've got all this wrinkly skin. But I do wear long sleeves at times for that very reason.

*In the first issue for 1993 of* Lysistra, *the magazine of Macquarie University women, there were some photographs of you naked, showing an older woman's body, which I found quite stunning. It was an acknowledgment that we do get old, and that age has its own beauty, that it's not ugly at all. Why did you do that?*

That's an interesting story. There was a group of, oh, ten women on the editorial collective: myself, and the other women were the usual twenties, and one was twenty-eight. We decided that we didn't want girly pictures, pretty little boobs and little bums; we wanted somebody older. So I was saying, 'Yes, we'll have to find somebody older,' and apparently they'd had this in their mind all along that they'd seen me as being the subject. And I said, well, yes I would. I had no awkwardness or embarrassment about it. In fact, they were greatly embarrassed by it more than I. They kept assuring me I'd be all right and I shouldn't worry, and sit down, and are you sure you're okay, and do you want a cup of tea? They were very protective and maternal of me. So I did it quite happily, but it was really an act of courage, knowing that everybody on university campus would see it and would know it was me. There was no head shot of course, just the body, but I imagine they'd have to know that's that old gal that hangs around with those radical women in the Women's Room. So, I did it for all of those reasons, that my young sisters should see how ageing looks, and that they must be aware that it's going to happen to them. For all of those reasons I became a centrefold of the student magazine.

*What sort of reaction have you had since?*
That's very interesting, Anne. None whatsoever. All my fears—I thought I'd be attacked verbally, and that youths would laugh and giggle and point at me. Nothing. Everybody feels unable to confront the reality. Some of the women that I've studied with and knew I was part of it, not even they came to me. They could have said, 'Hey, you've really done it this time and made a fool of yourself,' or alternatively they could have said, 'Oh that was pretty brave.' But they didn't say a damn word. I spoke to a few of them myself and, having prodded them, they said, 'Oh yeah that was terrific.' But, without prodding, none of them was able to come and say to me what they'd thought of it.

*I'm recalling now: my first reaction was amazement, because of the realisation that we don't ever see ourselves as we get older except in private. Older bodies are rarely displayed as public property, and so we can't celebrate getting old—whatever there is to celebrate about getting old—because it's bloody well hidden all the time. And so people are frightened of it or ashamed. You talked about wearing long sleeves over your wrinkly arms and thinking, 'Oh, my God.' Whereas, if it were more public, there would perhaps be less of this shame and rejection ... I don't know?*
Yeah, that what's I thought it would have done. Women would look at it and the men, too, and think this is the reality of their body a few years from now. Also, there's no sex about me as an old woman, and that's the main object why we photograph naked women—to show them as sex objects. So I don't look like a sexual being; just this great mountain of folding flesh and heavy, heavy breasts that are collapsing and folding down my chest. So I think that they don't see it as anything, except rather tragic, I imagine.

*That's one way of looking at it. The other way is to say: this is a body of a woman who has lived well and lived richly, and that body shows that. After all, we don't look at a tree that's old and collapsing, and think, what a huge, disgusting tree. We think, what a magnificent, immense old tree, don't we? Even a dog we look at and we say, 'Noble old dog.'*

I don't think we've got to noble old women, yet.

*As we get older, there seems to be an assumption that sexuality disappears. But it doesn't.*

No, no. It disappears because of the paucity of women your own age. But it doesn't disappear. One's needs and sexual urges are there, but they can't be utilised because there's no partnering available. There seems to be a great shortage of women of my age.

*In fact, the concept of older people having sexual feelings and being sexual beings is often made an object of ridicule.*

You see a lot of jokes about older people in sexual endeavour. You see cartoons of people sort of literally being propped up in the combat position, and a lot of jokes about the inability of the old to engage in sexual activity. But I don't think that's true. There might need to be some modification, of course, but the ability's there as indeed is the desire.

*So within you, do you feel still like a young person?*

Oh, I feel young, because I have body movement, and my head is active, and I move around and I meet people, and I do a lot of things. So I feel that this sort of activity and health should belong to a younger person. But it doesn't.

*A lot of people express extreme amazement at the fact that somehow or other they have arrived at old age.*

I was amazed when it happened to me. As I said earlier, it hit me when I was about fifty-five, and I had to accept that people viewed me as old. Indeed, it was amazing that they could dare to think that I was old when I knew I wasn't. I was active and busy and happy and healthy.

*Have you planned for your old age?*

Yes I have, very seriously. I think that must come from my good Catholic working-class background, the rainy-day theory. I started planning for these ageing years a long time ago, maybe when I was forty—but economic planning, not emotional. And because of my sexual preference, I knew that I was never going to have a man to 'care for me' and I would have to be dependent upon my own money for the rest of my life. I'm happy to say that I now have independence economically. I don't have to be beholden to the boys; I can be quite sassy and cheeky to them, because I don't have to buy their grace and favours or be polite to them.

*Margaret, talk a little bit about your childhood.*
Well, father was a public servant. He started off in the post office in the country town of Bega, far south coast. I remember him saying he was a horse-drawn postman. He wasn't the horse; he rode in a cart drawn by a horse, which was one of the first ones. Before that, they walked, and he would have walked miles before he was promoted to a horse. He stayed in the public service and went up the ladder and, in the end, he was internal auditor with one of the commonwealth departments. I know he had his own office when I went to visit him, so that impressed me. I gather he was quite important.

Cheerless, aloof, was the word I would have called him rather than being clever and astute. I don't have much memory of my father, really, other than his work.

*And your mother?*
My mother? Well, there, I have different memories. A girl always remembers her mother—

*You're smiling now; were they good memories?*
—They were, yes. I was smiling at that expression, 'A girl always remembers her mother.' Yes, she was a nice woman. I was very fond of her. When father died, she became ill—muscular dystrophy—and I nursed her, and that was a hard time. The brother and sister wanted out, so I was stuck (stuck indeed I was) with mother, caring for her. And then she went to hospital and died.

*How old were you?*
I was then thirty-five. She was always very gentle and very nice and very loving and ... and she was my friend.

*Was the Catholic church a significant part of your growing up?*
It was indeed. I was a born Catholic. By this I mean a 'real' Catholic, not a convert. It was in my blood, and the parents were, too. And the whole early memories of my youth were of the church, and the parish priest, and the monsignor, and the bishops, and those nuns, and the whole Catholic bit. My behaviour was dictated by the Catholic rules of the day. I was an obedient and dutiful child. I was clean, and I always had a handkerchief in my pocket. I never spoke unless spoken to, and we could display no emotion. That wasn't polite. I was kind to other little children, and I did the messages. I was the most obedient and appropriate Catholic child of the time, because that was what I was told to be.

I had no concept that there was any other way, because all the other dumb kids were equally as obedient and repressed. I guess I didn't realise all that until I left home on a working holiday when I was seventeen. And then I made certain observations, and left the church eventually—left it physically, that means. I don't go to mass, but I still say that it has got its hand around my throat and in my heart. Somehow, I still keep lapsing back to Catholic working-class values.

*Why did you leave school early?*
I would have had no choice. We all left school at fifteen, all the girls in my class, because that is 'what we did'. We had to get 'A Job.' I knew there was something called the university which some people went to, but it didn't occur to me. I wasn't given an option. I was told to go to the Public Service Board and there do an entrance examination, and become a clerk in the public service. That way, I would have security if I missed out on marriage; a permanent lifetime job in the public service as a spinster; and, when I retired, I would get this big superannuation, and my life would be made for me.

*And you accepted?*
Yes, I did. There was nothing that told me there was any other life. No friends, none of those evil nuns, no companions. There was nobody anywhere that made me think that I could have done anything else. And since all of the girls in my class scurried off and did the same thing, it clearly was what had to be done.

*But then you began to break away?*

Yes. With some of these same girlfriends, we went off on the working holiday—the working holiday which later was to continue on to England. But we got as far as Jervis Bay on the New South Wales south coast. We all became housemaid-waitresses in a ratty old guesthouse by the sea where we were abused by this owner of the guesthouse. We worked about twenty-four hours a day, but it was fun. We were away from mummy and daddy, we met boys, we learned how to drink, and how to kiss fellers, and nothing more. We learned all those gentle arts of flirtation of young Catholic ladies of the time.

*Was this a happy period?*

Oh, yes. I was having fun. I was out there in the world, and all the fellers and the dates, and the work and the sharing with all the women—there were four of us that went away together. Then I went up to the far north coast, Lismore, and then up to the Queensland Barrier Reef to work on one of the islands as a waitress again. I don't know how I managed to get away from home. I know there was some objection from the parents, but by then they must have deemed I was old enough to be independent and earn my own living.

*And then you had a baby?*

Yes I did, at age twenty-two. Once again, here comes the good old Catholic youth, that my mother had never explained any of this to me. You'd wonder how I got through Jervis Bay, kissing the boys and all. I knew there was something that they called, 'Down there', but all I knew was I wasn't going to have anything to do with it. And then finally this fellow came along who was nice and made all these promises that nothing would happen, 'Don't be silly, it'll be okay.' So because he said that it would be okay, I did—even though I knew that it was naughty. I'd been told that you didn't have sex before marriage. If you weren't a virgin you were never going to get a decent man to marry you, and then also you might get pregnant. But since this man said it was not possible, I did. I did 'Do It' and I did get pregnant. I can't even remember the act or if It was worth it. It must have been very brief and fleeting. So here I was pregnant and, of course, I couldn't tell 'my mummy and my daddy.' When I later thought about it, I suppose they were the cause in a sense, because of their Catholicism and their refusal to give me a chance by giving me any sex education.

So instead of saying, 'Well, righto, here you are, it's your fault,' and dumping it back on them—no, I went off on yet another working holiday to Queensland. It was very hard to find a job when I was so pregnant, but I found a live-in job with some old guy as his housekeeper. It was pretty hard, because he was an old fool, and I had no money and had to stay there. And then the time came, and I just rang up the ambulance and went off to the hospital. There again, even more ignorance. If I didn't know how to become pregnant, I certainly didn't know how to have a baby. I didn't know what they were doing with me: 'Turn over' and 'Do this.' I didn't even know how it would come out. It's amazing, this sort of ignorance. Eventually it must have come out, because then I had to sign a whole bunch of papers—which meant that it was gone.

*Did you hold the baby?*
Oh, no. Nothing like that was allowed. I had to get back to where I was staying. I had to get on to this old tram, which rattled and rattled and shook, and of course I was sore and bleeding and aching. I kept thinking it was a bitter twist on 'Streetcar Named Desire'. I had this old suitcase, and I had to drag myself and this suitcase home on the tram. So that was my adventure into motherhood.

*Did you cry when you got home?*
No, no, I don't think so. I was pretty tough.

*Did any friends know what was happening to you?*
Oh no, I couldn't tell anyone, 'cause they would tell mummy. So it was a secret.

*And what were the hospital people like to you?*
Oh, they were awful. In the fifties, it was the fallen woman syndrome: that if you were pregnant and you were unmarried, you were a slut or a whore, a cheap woman or a prostitute. They treated me without any consideration, and didn't speak to me. One consideration: they put me right up the far end of the ward in a bed, off on my own, so that when all the happy daddies and grannies and other kids would come in to see all the women with their little babies, I was up the end without a little baby. I secretly suspect they put me there to punish me.

*Have you grieved about this since?*

No, I haven't. A great many people would wish to have me grieve about it, but I try not to accept any grief at all. I'm quite dismissive of it. I'm only angry at that man who, who ... could treat another person in such an abominable way, it was ... very unfair of him. But I don't mourn the child. I don't, don't *wish* a child so... so I ... I lost nothing ... I wouldn't have wanted it—what would I do with a kid who'd now be forty and equipped with children, and possibly their children?

**You've never had any feeling later that you'd like to go back and find your son?**
No, only the anger at the father. And the anger at ... my inconvenience.

**What were you like as a child?**
I remember I was a shy, wispy, frightened little thing. I had very fine silky soft hair, which I still have. It used to hang all limp because it couldn't be curled or set up. I think I felt—and looked pretty well what I was—a silly little dopey Catholic kid.

**And when you were in your twenties, thirties?**
I dressed very conservatively at the time, and I wasn't a handsome woman or attractive one. That's all I can tell you about the twenties.

**Okay. Look back now on the period in your life when you felt you were at your peak.**
Always do the ones you like. That was when I met my partner, mid-sixties, this late-remembered one of twenty years' duration. I was very healthy and spunky and athletic, and I looked pretty sharp. I've got pictures of those times. I had red hair, and I was quite slim, and I had a really neat waist which I used to show off with great heavy leather belts on the top of my jeans, and I wore riding boots.

When I went to work I was more conservative. We had to wear dresses in those days, so I affected little skirts and little handbags and make-up. But in my private life I looked pretty sharp, like a real dyke, as in the role played in the sixties, like a young warrior woman. I was on top of the world. I had good jobs and income, and we lived a great life. We travelled a lot, we went clear around the world on one occasion of four months' vacation. We went to the States on vacation two or three times. I was in love and happy, fulfilled with my work and my relationship. And I looked spunky. That was my good time, Anne.

*When did you decide that you were homosexual?*
When a woman kissed me. I was on this ship travelling from Fort Everglades in Florida to Hamburg in Germany, and there was this woman—I can remember her name and everything about her—who kissed me. I know that's too simplistic, and it's been said by these same people who would have me grieve for that child, that there must have been more than just liking to be kissed by a woman instead of being kissed by a man. But again, I think it's as simple as that. I preferred women.

*In some of your writing you have made the observation that, had you known more then, maybe you would not have made that choice to be lesbian—because of the alienation and the loneliness that you've sometimes felt since then. That suggests that for you there was a matter of choice?*
Oh, yes. I could have repelled Brigetta and gone off with the ship's engineer. But I must have *preferred* her company, and then I didn't ever continue with men. I came back to Australia as, I thought, the only lesbian in the world, and somehow had to manage to live when there were no other lesbians in Sydney forty years ago. That was a lonely time, knowing that I had this ... affliction, this ... state.

*Is that how you saw it?*
Yes, because at the time it was written about very badly. There was no joy in it, and we were evil women. So I didn't see it as anything good that had come upon me. Then the woman that I worked with in an office ... I'm pausing here; I don't know how to put this ... Yes, I seduced her; that was it. She was a woman fifteen years younger, fortuitously, because then we could hide it as Margaret and her little friend Jann. So we hid that for a few years, then we decided we'd get out of town, because it was looking a bit awkward. So we decided on yet another working holiday. Working holidays got me in and out of so much trouble! Off we went back to the States again. And there it happened, there were lesbians and lesbian magazines, and gay bars and a gay community in San Francisco. So that was rather pleasing, to see that there were other people and it was okay. We stayed there until we ran out of visas, came back home to Australia, and set up two separate households.

And then Jann married, in the endeavour of being seen to go out with men. It was the glorious Vietnam war, R and R days, and these American servicemen came to Australia. We went to some of their cocktail parties simply because there was free grog. They were provided by the American Embassy: bring the women, give them free grog, and they can act as hostesses to our boys. So Jann met this ... paid killer, who was a lieutenant commander in the Navy and ... married him. And that was really grieving. She went back to the States. She lives now in Seattle, Washington, with this man who ended up a full commander in the Navy. She's rich. She's got two motor cars and a kid that has got braces on its teeth, and she claims that she never told Gerry about her earlier fall from grace. But I believe that she has, because he never receives me very warmly.

*When you think about being a lesbian, you used the word 'affliction' earlier—what do you think about it now?*

I wouldn't use the word 'affliction'. That was a word of the time. I'm sure the church and medicine at the time called it 'affliction', because we had aversion therapy in those times to get rid of it. No, I'd call it now ... disaccommodating that ... I am a lesbian at sixty-six. There is no companionship for a lesbian of my age. And having—

*Forgive me interrupting. Why is it any worse for a lesbian at your age than for a heterosexual woman at your age who's on her own?*

I have a theory that the heterosexual woman on her own is part of the general community. She has some neighbours; she has some friends; she was likely married, so she's got some children and grandchildren. She's a pensioner, she belongs to the club, they play bowls, they sit on the bus seats and engage each other in conversation. I've lived in a lesbian ghetto for most of my life, amongst lesbians only. I call my politics 'separatist' in that I don't have any male contacts and don't wish to converse with them even. So I've put myself in this ghetto of my own making. I only get out of it to speak to lesbian women and feminist women, and there are very few of them of sixty-plus. I say that my loneliness is because of the narrowness of my choice of companions.

*Why have you done this?*

Why? I think it was the time when the women's movement arrived in Australia, in the late sixties. We lived in a women's community. There were so many of us, they were such heady and exciting days. We were involved in political actions and meetings and groups, and our world was composed of women. So, having started that way, that there were no men involved, that they were the enemy, according to our theory, I just didn't fall into that company. And so I went on, year after year, until I entered into my last and final relationship of twenty years' duration. But her friends and my friends were women only. It was inconceivable that we could go out to dinner with a couple of fellows and find as much company or interest in them as we would with two sisters. It came upon itself by preference. I enjoy women's company, and women's excitement, and women's stimulation and support, and women's politics, and women's sexuality. I can't get out of it, now, because I have nothing in common with most women my age. Women of my age are grandmothers, are married women. They aren't political. I find it difficult speaking to them or understanding how they function— just as they would find it difficult understanding how I function.

*Tell me about 'The Old Lesbian Organising Committee'.*

Oh, this is a group in the United States. We'd like to use the same idea here in Australia. One of the purposes would be to confront ageism within our own lesbian community and in the larger community— analyse our experiences of ageism, develop educational material. But we see it as a support group of old dykes, because our interests are different from our younger sisters.

For instance, it is ageist when 'old' is used in a derogatory manner and 'young' is used as a compliment. And another one: when you automatically expect an old lesbian to share her financial resources and energy with you. And this is a good one: an old lesbian's anger is trivialised as 'feisty'. Another one: when you automatically assume that an old lesbian is asexual. And here: an outspoken old lesbian is described as 'complaining', 'crotchety', or 'difficult'; younger people don't necessarily accept that you're being political and you want to be heard. They will just call you 'an old bag', 'an old crochety', or 'an old complainer'.

*Do you think that there is less ageism in other societies, even societies that are in some ways similar to ours? Say, America?*

I don't find it as bad there at all, particularly in restaurants and diners and these little coffee bars where the waiter persons are women, old women, and they're really characters. They laugh, and they talk, and they call everyone 'honey', and they have purple or red hair. They wear these great big heavy rubber shoes that waiters wear. You see them everywhere, but particularly in these jobs. I've wondered why: is it that young women don't want to work in these jobs which are pretty arduous and boring? Or is it that management see that old women are good for that sort of work—they're warming and they're welcoming, they care for people and look after them well, they're more interested in work, and they take their responsibilities more seriously. You see them in other areas, driving the public transport, and in offices all the time when you go to do business there.

*Do you feel that as you've got older you are able to be more yourself?*
Yes, that's another thing that comes with ageing: you get away with more. So if I do something really wild, people seem to tolerate it by just thinking, 'Well, she *must* be an eccentric, or she wouldn't dare say this, or do this, or dress like that.' I find that I can say what I want and do as I wish because of my economic independence, and that they—the boys—can't touch me.

*Are there stereotypes of an old lesbian which are different from stereotypes of an old heterosexual person—an old hetero?*
[Laughs] An old hetero. Well, yes, the other two 65-year-old dyke women I know look a bit like me. We don't dress as conservatively as 68-year-old grannies. And I think we're identifiable. Women tell me that I'm identifiable, that I look like a dyke. So that's something to be proud of. That's what it cost me to get here. I still wear it, I'm known as a dyke, and that pleases me.

*The word 'dyke', is that something that pleases you?*
Oh yes, I like that word. It was a word of abuse, as was 'nigger'; you know, American blacks now call themselves this quite fondly. We've taken it back and glorified it, and politicised lesbians call themselves 'dykes'. There's no other word. We don't even use the word 'lesbian' necessarily. It's 'dyke'.

*What made you become politicised?*
Elizabeth Reid, who was Whitlam's adviser on Women's Affairs in 1975, had organised this great conference in Canberra, 'Women and Labor'. We went to that, and after all those sessions and workshops and sharing

and talking, we came away at the end of ten days committed to being politicised feminists.

*And you've remained politicised?*
I have, yes. There's no one word for what the women's movement wants. We would wish to be treated not as a separate second sex, less equal. We would wish to have more women representing us in all areas of government and legislation. We wish to have more equal representation.

*Do you feel there have been improvements in the last ten, fifteen years?*
Oh, indeed, I've certainly seen them since those halcyon days of Whitlam in Canberra. There have been a great many improvements for women in their working conditions, and in political ways, and in acceptance by the community of women as such. There are things that have only happened because women have fought for them. The young women aren't as political, because they think it's all been done. But they perhaps are not aware of the battles; they weren't present, they aren't necessarily written up, so they don't know what we really *did* for them. They just come along, and there it is, and they take it.

*Do you feel that women's attitudes to you are different from male attitudes? Are they kinder towards women who are older?*
Yes, I believe that they are. As I'm travelling about doing my business, on the buses or whatever, a woman would give a smile or give a seat or pass a greeting with you. Whereas men rarely do. So I think that particularly women of my age will give one of these conspiratorial little smiles at you as if they're saying, 'Oh yes, we know, we're old. We know what it's like.'

*How do you feel about moving into your seventies?*
I feel bad. There's only the university between me and isolation. It's getting more difficult to sustain myself, so I guess when I'm in my seventies it'll really be tough.

*Have you any idea what might help you?*
No. I don't know what would help me, other than society changing its attitudes and being nicer to the aged. Then I'd feel fine. But I'm also

in fear of being this age, and living in my house as I do quite independently. I'll come to the point where I'll need to have care. That's a word for going into one of those houses where people go to wait to die. I feel quite depressed about that, because again I'll be with these same women that I've never been with anywhere in my life—old women of seventy-five, eighty—who've all married, all been grandmothers, had children. I'll have nothing to share with them.

We all make the jokes about the old dykes' home. Most of the women that I grew up with in the women's movement, the old sister warriors, we keep talking about the old dykes' home, but all of us are reluctant to do it. We want to hang on to our homes and our privacy and our independence and our health for as long as we can. No one wants to start. If I, for instance, sold my house and said, 'All right, we've got two hundred and fifty thousand dollars. You sell yours, Mary'—there's another, you know, four houses—we'd have a million dollars! We could buy a grand house which would still maintain our independence and privacy, but have a common meeting-area where we'd come together whenever we wanted to. Nobody's done it. But I have some hope that we may come to that. Then I could live with four great old warrior women of seventy. That'd be good, wouldn't it?

*Or eighty? Or ninety?*

Yes, or ninety. And we'd have these young spunky dykes who'd be the nurses and carers and the chauffeurs.

*Are you frightened of dying?*

No, no. That'd be my way out. At last I've got away from that Catholic myth. I have no belief in an afterlife or a heaven or a hell. When I die I merely die, and my body's disposed of.

*How would you like to be remembered?*

As a woman warrior.

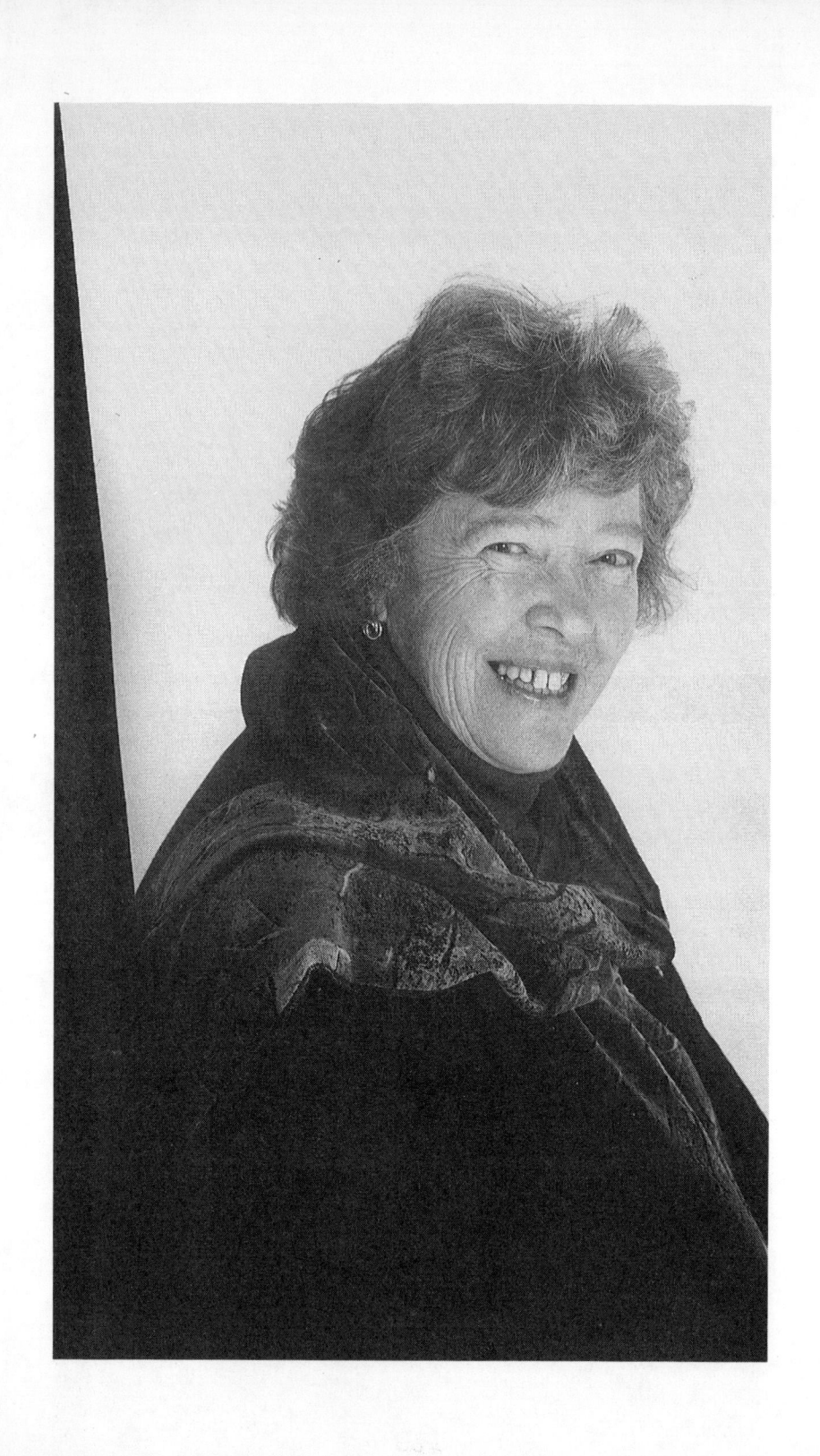

# Delys Sargeant
## *No wigs for our pubes*

Delys Sargeant, who was born in Toodyay, Western Australia in November 1927, is a challenging and highly regarded educator in the field of sexuality and human relationships. Her first research was into the reproductive cycle of the West Australian crayfish, which she says enabled her to experience the privilege of eating her way through her data.

She founded the Social Biology Resources Centre in Melbourne in 1973, and was its director until 1992. The Centre has educated thousands of health, welfare, and education workers across Australia, and has taken major initiatives in the integration of people with disabilities in training and employment. At one period, the Centre attracted strong hostility from groups which took a reactionary stance towards sexuality education in schools. To safeguard the Centre's work, Delys took successful legal action through the Supreme Court in 1979.

Delys Sargeant has served on a number of major state and federal enquiries and advisory groups; and, for her pioneering community-health work, she was awarded membership of the Order of Australia in 1993. She is married, has three adult children, and lives in Victoria.

Something that's special about being older is having a clearer acceptance of time. When I was younger, I carried many more 'shoulds' and 'musts' about tasks, and about how I used time. I was much more anxious about a lot of things. Nowadays, I know more about what to expect, and what actions are needed to be 'safe.' I remember vividly my first experience of seeing ocean waves when I was a young child; of making friends as an adolescent; of new parenting. All these experiences developed intuitive learning, most of which is so unconscious that you tend to think that you were born with these instincts for knowing what is safe, what are the limits to set, and what are the risks you can take. Also, I know how to use my 'intuitings'—how to develop and call on friends.

*Are friends important to you?*

Yes, very. Most of my early life I was scared witless that I would never be able to make friends. I grew up in a fairly isolated farming community. There were four children in our family, and we attended a primary school of only nine children, so we didn't get too much opportunity to test out making friends with our own age group. When I went to boarding-school at the age of twelve, I was desperately worried at my lack of friendship-making skills.

*Did you have a privileged childhood?*

Oh, yes. I was the first born of parents who showed their love for each other and to me and my brothers, and I was a loved grandchild. I know my mother and father had enormous confidence, which I 'caught' from them, that I was going to be not just a goody-goody, but a special girl in some way.

I always felt I had a right to be myself and, for a girl in that country district, that was pretty unusual in the thirties and forties. Women friends and relatives criticised my mother for *letting* me go away to school and to university. Girls were expected to be companions to their mothers, helping with all the tasks of farmers' wives—like providing nice afternoon teas when the accountant came round, and food and flowers in the local hall for the various functions, and meeting all those domestic and social commitments that were expected of women on the land.

*Isn't this interesting? I'm sure if I'd asked many people whether their childhood was privileged, their replies would have been in economic terms. Your response was about emotions. But in an economic sense, was it privileged?*

Oh no, it wasn't economically privileged at all, because my parents married in 1926, and I was born early in the Depression. They started off a farm with debt, and incurred a great deal more debt in those years before the war. I don't ever recall feeling that we were deprived, but I know that my parents were financially very worried. I can recall my father would anxiously switch on the wireless to check the price of wheat. Money was not available, and we had very few books. I remember the agony of excitement when the box of library books arrived on the train once every two months.

My privilege was that my parents provided an emotional security. They would disagree, and we could see them argue, but there was never any violence. There was a lot of talking and discussion and of sharing with us the things they both enjoyed. My mother was a very individual person, and I had a grandmother who was an extremely strong-willed matriarch. So these two women were influential in my early understanding of 'women's power.' My father was an affectionate, dominant, *interested* person; and my very gentle grandfather, a dignified, quiet, almost reclusive man who ultimately got Parkinson's disease—so I saw him in his later years in a very debilitated state of dependency.

My grandmother must have had a pretty hard time in opening up their property at the turn of the century. She used to help log and remove trees, and she established the Country Women's Association in Bolgart in Western Australia in 1920, apparently against quite a lot of opposition from the men in the district. She was a prime mover in the building of the local church, started the Mother's Union, the tennis club, and the golf club, the whole lot.

*How important are the memories of your grandmother?*

You'll die when I tell you, but a strong memory is of her smell—she was a smelly old lady.

*Was she smelly because she was old, or was she smelly anyway?*

No, she was smelly because she was incontinent. Maybe she was always a bit smelly but it became a worse smell as she got older. I used to loathe going into her bedroom, because she always had a chamber pot under the bed, and her body seemed to reek of urine. I've always been smell-conscious. I didn't like her terribly much, but I loved her.

*What did you love about her if you didn't like her?*

Her constancy. She was absolutely reliable. I knew that the love she gave me was unconditional, and that I was her grand-daughter. So there was no lack of identity, no lack of being part of the family. But she was not the sort of person that I could ever have talked with as a youngster, and she was a bit fearsome in the way she was so definite in her opinions. I talked with my grandfather's sister, who was of the same age group. She was a wonderful woman. She was big, and I remember as a little child loving the surety of somehow being under*neath* her. I could look up over her tummy.

Although she was uneducated, I always had a sense of her dignity and her intelligence: there was something about the way she sat and her composure. She listened with her whole body, so she was a very special older person. What worried me about her as she got older was her intellectual rigidity, and it was a little bit the same with my grandmother. I tended to believe this is what happens to you as you get older, and this has been a deeply buried anxiety about being older until relatively recently. I have reflected on what old age meant to these two women who saw such changes in their life times, and I do wish I could talk to them now.

*What is it that you think you might watch out for, when you are old?*

Well, I certainly don't want to be a smelly old lady! I do have some incontinence, so I am anxious to deal effectively with that. I don't think I've got much to worry about being mentally rigid, because I've had such an ongoing and extraordinary educational opportunity to learn, and this tends to offset rigidity. There have been times when I get very anxious by a lack of memory and I think, 'Oh-oh, here it starts!' A big thing that scares me about being old is that the words won't come and my ideas won't flow, won't go on wings.

*When you say 'worries you', to what extent does it worry you? Do you lie awake at night worrying?*

No. When it happens I start to get reflective, and I try to avoid making decisions if I am tired. I've learned that when I *am* feeling tired, I need to acknowledge it. I find it very important to have more restorative time, time to sit quietly.

*Okay, so how are you reacting to this need to re-pace your life? With*

*impatience, or with interest?*
Oh, it's very much with interest. It's like being intrigued with a new palette, looking at the different colours and then creating wonderful new blends. Somebody asked me the other day what were some of the special things about growing older. And, quick as a flash, I said, 'Lying awake in the morning and knowing that there's no panic. That I can elect to read or to listen to the radio, or shut my eyes and go to sleep again.' There are very few times when I now commit myself to early-morning meetings. So that's a change in my life. I find I'm sleeping better. I'm sleeping 'clean', which means that my stress levels are much lower than they were even twelve months ago.

I'm quite intrigued at the way in which my body is happily adjusting to the lesser demands placed on it. I'm still using my brain as actively as before, but I don't have anything like the same demands of administration and organisational pressure. I have control over when I talk to people at home, because I have an answering machine. And there are all sorts of ways in which I'm actually pacing my time and my tasks, and really enjoying it. But I am intrigued that I am also feeling a sense of loss because I have less informal contact with people, more isolated time, less 'stuff' passing over the desk, and I'm not so *included*.

*What about the process of biological change?*
This has been going on for as long as I can remember, and it's not a special issue in my sixties. I don't like my weight; I don't like my fat much. I had a biopsy some years ago, and had a benign lump removed from under my arm. I've noticed that it's all fattened up again, so it's a fair chance that the same lump has grown again. I thought yesterday morning about the discomfort I have with such full breasts, so if there is a new lump and it needs to be removed, I might actually ask whether my breasts could be reduced at the same time. You know what a coward I am about 'elective' surgery, but the discomfort of carrying heavy breasts seems to be increasing, and I know they are likely to get still bigger as I age further.

And there's the great big fat pad on my abdomen that just doesn't want to go. It seems very attached to me! I find the fat distributed on my body is unattractive, and a bloody nuisance. I can't do up my shoelaces as easily as I did [laughs]. I need to lose weight, and get back to some regular exercise. It's not beyond me; it's a matter of adjusting my life.

*What about your appearance?*

Don't like my neck. I investigated what was involved with a plastic surgeon, and also I had seen the film, *Daisy has a Face Lift*. It's a repelling procedure and, given the risks, even though low, of death or disablement from thromboses, it seems foolish to be electively mutilated. It seems that the people who are important to me love me regardless of my neck. It's *me* that doesn't like it. And since I don't have to look at myself all that often, it struck me that, if other people can bear the sight of me, well then what's the point? I was surprised that my children were so disturbed by the idea of my having plastic surgery. Our families seem to get used to our physical changes rather more readily than we do!

*As you've got older—*

I'm nearly beyond the third age.

*— has this changed the nature of your relationship with John, your husband?*

Yes. It has gained. I think this is partly due to the changes in his work life. Since he has released himself from a work environment, which for most of his adult life was clearly incredibly stressful, he has changed much more than I have with my change of occupation. He's happy and more creative and less intense. When he does get stressed, he shows little snatches of what he used to be like, and that's a real shock. Recently I said to him I thought we should go away for a holiday, and he said, 'What do you mean, a holiday? I'm *on* a holiday all the time.' So I suggested we go away for two weeks *work*!

I was afraid there may be difficulties in our relationship after I left the Centre, and I think maybe John assumed that I would be a regular farm worker, being available to prune his grape vines. Ever since I've come back from Europe he's recognised that his fantasies of me and retirement weren't reality. My 'head' work and engagement with people continues to be very important to me. John has become much more involved in my work than he ever was, since I now don't have secretarial back-up, and people ring me at home. He takes messages, and talks to people who contact me at the farm, and it is good to have him interested in what I would normally have thought too trivial to discuss. It balances out my involvement in his viticulture and wine production.

Our adjustment has been pretty smooth. We've always been

independent, yet co-workers, and we respect that in each other. Our relationship has deepened, and our times of fun together have increased, while the intensities of parenting are very reduced. Sure, there will always be something that we may disagree or be anxious about in the lives of our adult children—but this older stage of life seems just so much easier for us as parents. It gives us more free time together, yet always with the pleasures associated with having adult children and with grandparenting. It's calmer, and there's more time to 'be'.

*Have people's attitudes towards you changed?*
Yes. It's interesting the number of people who say, 'Oh, now that you've retired.' Or they say, 'Is that how old you are? I'd no idea!' There's still strong negative stereotyping about being over sixty-five. I've attempted, in my professional life, to use myself as a model of an older woman who feels very independent, vigorous, free-thinking, change-focussed, exploratory, and risk-taking. And sometimes it's great fun to challenge stereotypes that people are obviously holding. Over the last few years, when work was very stressful and people would comment, 'Oh, you do look tired,' I would suddenly think, 'Oh God, my lines must be showing' or 'It's my turkey neck.' In other words, I was quick to put bad stuff on myself. The ease with which I upheld my own negative views of ageing sometimes concerned me.

To resist this, and to acknowledge that it required new coping skills, I chose self-talk. I would say, 'Well, it's surprising that I don't look more tired, given what I'm doing.' I've actively worked on rephrasing and reframing my thoughts of myself. It takes a lot of effort to reject negative stereotypes commonly held in society—that older women are forgetful, stupid, irresponsible, unreliable, emotional. All those self-discounts are so readily applied when we get caught short, and when we are surrounded by younger people who can show just the same behaviours.

*Have you changed the way you dress?*
Yes. I had a wonderful time in Europe immediately after I retired. It gave me space between living with people who knew me well, and working and living with people that did not. I enjoyed testing out different ways of dressing as a 'new old' woman—small things, like wearing flat shoes pretty well all the time, while over here I've always enjoyed a higher heel. So, when I was working in Copenhagen for the

World Health Organisation, I wore new-style hats. I've worn hats pretty well consistently since my return. Something about wearing a hat gives me a feeling of risk-taking, and makes me feel really good. I think an older woman can do more semi-outrageous things because of the stereotypes which associate being older with eccentricity. I'm a much calmer and more confident person in many ways, and my dress reflects this.

**What else do you want to do that's outrageous?**
Apart from hats? Well, I only started skinny-dipping when I was around about fifty; and that's a long time to always wear bloody bathers, isn't it? I feel quite confident now to float around naked in the swimming pool, and it's such a lovely, free feeling. It really is crazy that, with my old, fatter, more floppy body, I'm much better about getting into the pool without any clothes on than twenty years ago, when I couldn't overcome my modesty to do so with a much trimmer body.

Other outrageous things? I'm not a person that needs to do physically exhilarating things like bungy jumping, and what I would classify as physical risk-taking. My joints aren't good, so I'm not going to put them at risk. I did that for long enough while I was skiing. So I'm cautious about doing things that might hurt me, because I really want to keep my mobility. I *would* like to go hot-air ballooning. My risk-taking is more in my thinking, and also in taking up creative activities. I'm certainly going to have a go at ceramics. I'm doing pastel work; and I'm going to try pastels on fabric, in the Japanese style of unrolling them. It's not really risk-taking: it's assigning more time and value for creative playing.

**Much earlier, you were talking about memories of your grandmother and the fact that she was incontinent—is this still a fear for you?**
Oh yes, because I do leak. My fear is lack of control and what this may lead to if I am limited in where I live, or require care, as my mother and mother-in-law and grandmothers did in their late lives. Incontinence is still a major deciding factor in whether people require institutional care. It's a simple condition which is used as a biological trigger to a whole social world which I would not want. So I hope my bladder doesn't lead me into a nursing home!

**So what are you going to do to help prevent that?**
Get myself into a better physical state, and know that as long as my

head works I can handle my environment. If my head doesn't work, I guess there's nothing much I can do about it. My family might want to 'unload' me at that point! But, you know, it's the unknown—how far you can actually manage your life and keep control over it.

*Would you ever contemplate killing yourself?*
I have once, so I know the feeling. It was one night, two weeks after our first born, our little two-and-a-half-year-old daughter had been buried. My parents had returned to West Australia, and John had not yet come home from his first day back at work. It was dusk, and Pippa's room was just so quiet. The whole house was empty and still. I was absolutely empty, and the stillness in me was a deep ... deep ... very deep chill. I was outside of me. I had joined Pippa, and we were looking down on the physical me. We were beside 'me' and yet inside 'me' at the same time. It was the most apart and serenely separated experience I think I have ever had. I recall thinking, 'I don't need to be "in me" any more.' I didn't actually attempt suicide; I think I was prevented from even exploring that by an unexpected visit from an immediate neighbour. I don't know what I would have done if she had not come at that time. I probably would have returned to a reality before the actuality, because I do very much like being alive.

I know my mother tried to commit suicide. She was a very full and creative person with an enormously exciting personality, until she had a series of strokes. She now couldn't speak and she couldn't do anything for herself. My father found her sitting in the wheelchair out in the garden where he had placed her, and she was trying to hit her own head with a stone which she had somehow been somehow able to reach. I know she didn't want to live, yet she was outside any capacity to do anything about that choice. I hope I'm never ever in that position.

*Would you kill yourself, though? If you knew you were going to be in that position, and you had the capacity to end your life?*
I haven't undone the plastic cover of that book—I've forgotten the author—which gives people clues about how to do that. I will read it some time, to know more. I would be very unhappy about anything which left someone else with discomfort as a consequence of any deliberate action. It would need to be very clearly understood by John that it was my choice and not his, and not because of him. I think I would make sure that it wasn't messy, and that it was effective. I sincerely

hope I won't need to make such a decision. I'm not in favour of people setting up their grand moment with all their family gathered round them while they snuff themselves!

*Why not?*

Because it may be nice for the person who's going, but what about the people who are living? I think we're all separate links in the chain of society, and that no man is an island. So I'm opposed to what I see as the ultimate self-focussed grand moment of choice.

*Do you think it should be at least not a crime?*

Oh yes. I can't see any point in seeing suicide as a crime at any age. If you want to do it, you want to do it. It's your life. I think it's a crime if you involve others. So it would be an immorality if, by attempting to do yourself in, you involved another person in some criminal way.

*As we've been talking about this—and obviously we're not exactly talking about a happy subject—your face started to look bleak. What was going on?*

I was recalling my daughter's death, and I was very sad. Also, I feel sad to know my mother felt like that at the end of her life. The need to *end* a life is so different from choosing the time to live. If you need to choose the time to end, it normally means that things are pretty intolerable and insufferable. So there's a deep sadness about that part of the human condition [pauses].

*Another area that's often a taboo is sex and sexuality.*

Yes. And although many taboos have been ostensibly overthrown, there continues to be much energy and interest in the subject! With all the oversexualising of our society, I am amazed that I still get almost daily requests around issues of sexuality from people who are working in the health and caring professions, and sometimes the media. I have recently focussed more on the health of older people, particularly older women. It is my aim to achieve significant changes in the way professionals, friends, and carers relate to older women and men about their sexual intimacies and concerns.

*Is there an assumption that as you get older you are no longer a sexual human being?*

Sure. Someone reported a young psychologist asking, 'Do you think *she* still does *it* at her age?' The consequences of such thinking is that if older people move to single beds they are often assumed to be 'not up to it' any more—rather than that they may be sleeping apart because of snoring, farting, or arthritis! People's intimacy patterns and idiosyncrasies are scrutinised and judged, even by family members, particularly if they need any special care. And in institutional care, older people tend to be infantilised and patronised.

I'm also interested in how older people who really want sexual intimacy manage to negotiate it. I've been told by some women in their late seventies how disgusted they are to see groups of women sitting in a hotel, looking longingly at any man that goes past on the way to the pokie machines. And that they'll drink more than they need while they're trying to be friendly to a sole feller that goes by. In other words, there's a lack of availability of unattached older men for women who stereotypically feel that to validate themselves they need to attract a man.

Opportunities for older women to have a new male partner are very limited in our society, and they become vulnerable to exploitation and to discounts from other women. There are certainly many older women who've had a great deal of discomfort in penetrative sex, and who are more likely than today's forty-year-olds to have been fairly ignorant when they were young, and perhaps have less experience of men other than their husbands. These women are often mightily relieved to support the myth that as you grow older you don't need sex. They say things like, 'Thank God I don't have to be bothered with *that* any more.' It's a real sadness to think that people see 'that' as being sexual. We don't talk enough about flirting; we don't talk enough about the loss of flirtatious opportunities for older men and women when they leave work—sexually validating and affirming experiences which were fun. When older people are seeking new partnerships, but poverty or disablement or distance limits their opportunities, then their sexual health is reduced.

***What sort of observations have you made about your own sexuality?***
I have changed physically in that, during arousal, I don't have the same sensations of pelvic change that I experienced when I was younger. But that can be accommodated. It's like saying, 'Oh well, my pubic hair's got thinner, and so I'll have to wear a wig for my pubes' [laughter].

I guess men have got something to tether a wig to! *No Wigs for Our Pubes*—what a title that would make for a book about sexuality and ageing!

It's those sort of body changes which play a minor part in the being of an older woman. But they are really very minor. I enjoy my older womanness. I enjoy my fun. I find that people that I like and love show me quite enough response to satisfy all my needs for social affirmation as a woman. I have a great deal of confidence in my marital relationship. Sometimes I say to John, 'We must be the most boring people if we really are interested and comfortable and having fun with each other after forty years.'

*Do you worry about death?*

I've undertaken a great deal more study of pain management than of death. I acknowledge that I may well arrive in a situation where I'm out of control of me, and experiencing pain. I don't like pain. I've had some circumstances where I've been very pained (bodily pained not mentally), and I don't want my death to be painful. But death is a part of what we are, so I don't fear it. I only would feel saddened if it was messy, both for me and for my loved ones.

*Have you any thoughts or philosophy about what happens after, if anything?*

For me, I don't think there will be a life afterwards. I have a strong philosophy that I am going to be spiritually alive as long as people remember me. I still remember very clearly people who have been very dear to me, and who have died. I really feel they're not dead. Sometimes, I almost hear them speaking to me. I think it was Dylan Thomas whose dead barmaid, Rosie Probert, used to say: 'Remember me, boys, I'm dying'. She wanted to stay alive through the memories of people who had known her. If people remember me, then that will be my hereafter.

*And how would you like them to remember you?*

As a loving and interesting person who was valued for my essence, and for having in some way contributed to the quality of their lives. I've been interested in reading recently about the different ways in which some men and women have anticipated their death. It seems that many men have a very instrumental view, like a tunnel or a door or a curtain through which they pass—something that's quite tangible. While many women have a perception of movement, of wind, of sound, and wings, or something making noise that's involved with wind. It really intrigued me, the notion that there might be a gender difference in the experience of transition into death. I wondered how much cultural variation there may be in this.

I believe that I have a very strong kinship with what I understand of Aboriginality, and that notion of a spiritual continuity with land—like the movement of tornadoes where the soil and the air and the sky are all in continuum: where there's no differentiation, no boundary between the solid and the not so solid. At one stage, I could think about literally sleeping on for ever. I think of what happens when I'm going into anaesthetic, and it's usually flashes of visual imagery and sounds. I guess it would depend on what was precipitating death. But even with sudden deaths—like from a massive heart attack—you still have seconds of consciousness that you're changing. So I hope my death moments will be interesting and confident. I hope that my mind will be able to enjoy those split-second visions of what has mattered in my living. And I hope that my death will be really important for those I love and who love me.

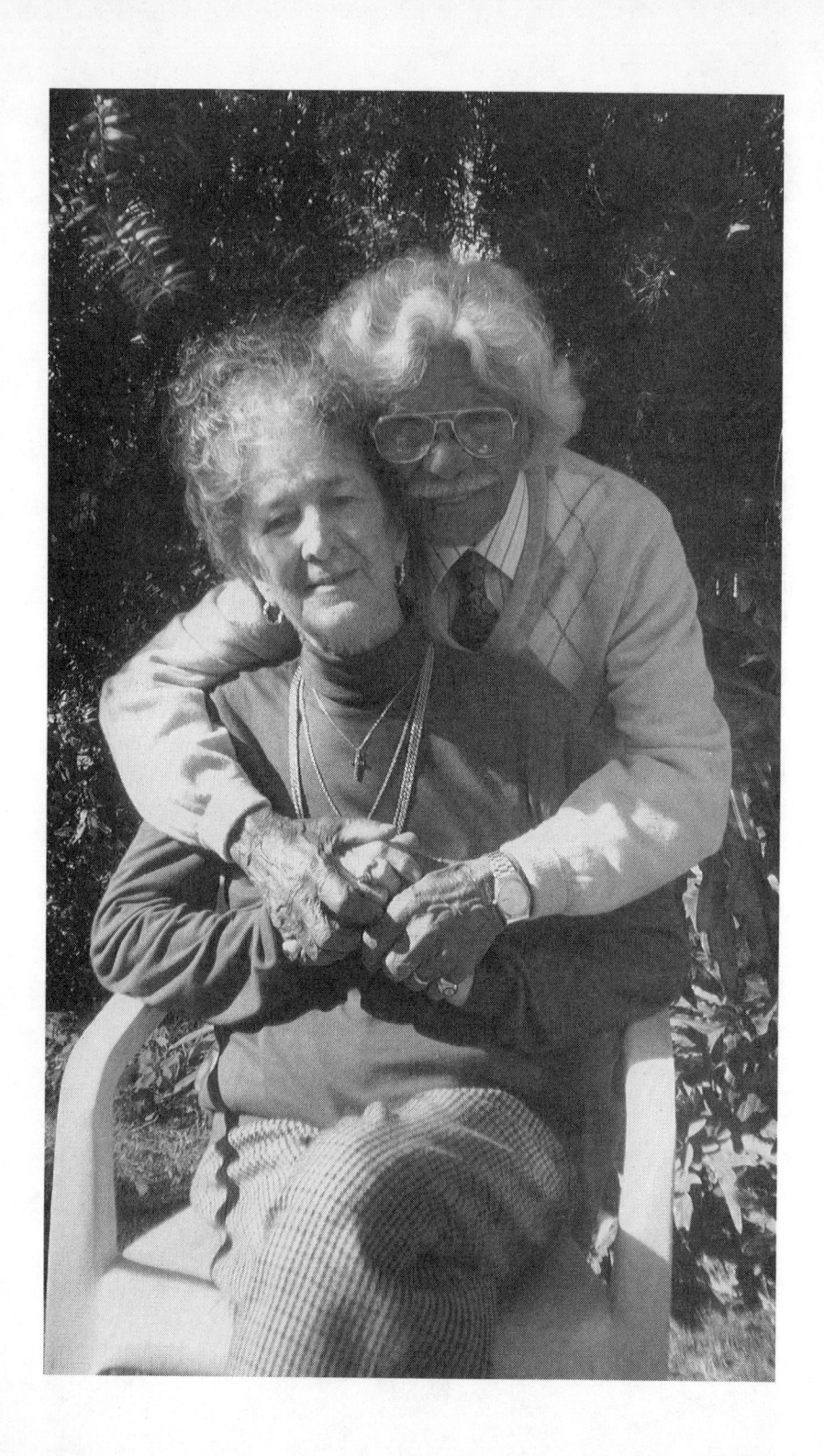

# Neville and Heather Bonner
*At the top of the mountain*

Neville Bonner, first Aborigine to be elected to the federal parliament, was born in Tweed Heads, New South Wales on 28 March 1922. Neville Bonner grew up knowing poverty, hunger, and discrimination. When he was thirteen, his mother died and he moved to Beaudesert, where he received his only formal schooling—for one year. He worked as a bush labourer, stockman, and carpenter before living for fifteen years on Palm Island near Cairns, where he became assistant overseer of the Aboriginal settlement.

Bonner then managed a Queensland dairy farm, worked for the Brisbane City Council, began his own business manufacturing boomerangs, joined the Liberal Party in 1967, and became a Queensland Liberal Party senator from 1971 to 1983. He was a board director of the Australian Broadcasting Corporation from 1983–91, and was made an officer of the Order of Australia in 1984.

Today, Neville Bonner maintains a strong involvement with numerous committees, including twenty years active campaigning for World Vision. He gives as his recreations golf, reading, and country music. His first wife, Mona, died in 1969, and he married Heather (born in 1923) three years later. Between them they have eight children, twenty-eight grandchildren and twenty-four great grandchildren.

If I go back to my early days as a young man, what I saw happen in non-Aboriginal communities towards the aged disgusted me. They left their old people living on their own, or they put them in a home. We don't do that. We take care of our aged. We love and admire and respect them, and that really and truly is one of the basic elements of Aboriginal culture.

Heather: No matter which section of the Aboriginal community we visit, Neville is Ol'man or Ol'fellow, and that's the highest regard. If I am accompanying Neville, I am Ol'lady or Ol'grandma or Ol'aunty. Neville can travel around Australia or overseas, and if I'm home alone, no Murri (we belong to the Murri community) would come around the house and cause a fuss, because Ol'man is away. 'Don't worry Ol'lady.' Even when Ol'man's home: 'Oh no, you don't go to Ol'man's house and cause a fuss.' Murris, who would 'murmur murmur murmur' behind Neville's back, change the moment he appears on the scene: 'Oh no, that's Ol'man, eh ... don't do that to Ol'man ... look, Ol'man's here, eh.' Now we don't have that in our culture. By and large, we have lost respect for our elderly people. That's something I've learned from the Aboriginal culture—the great respect for older people and their wisdom and experience of living.

I am so privileged to be getting older in this culture. I come back to this feeling of safety and caring. In the city where we live, or any city which we happened to be visiting, if we lost all our money or we had no food, we'd go to the nearest Aboriginal home, and they'd share their last bit of food with us. You can't say that about the white culture.

*Is that going to last, do you think?*

Heather: It will be some generations, but I do think ultimately it will die out. However, there is more Aborigine within the Aborigine than the Aborigine lets on. An Aborigine within his or her home is an Aborigine, and so are the children. In the home a Murri is a Murri is a Murri. You just don't show it off to the white person.

Neville: We have learned from bitter experience that you don't show your Aboriginality in the presence of non-Aboriginal people—because if you do, then you're branded straight away. You're a black, you're a boong, you're an abo. You've got to put on a facade as though you're one of the general community. And so we withdraw: we are Murris amongst Murris, we are Australians amongst whites.

*What sort of things might you do or say amongst yourselves?*
Neville: Speech, mannerisms, all sorts of things. Our humour, for instance. When Heather and I have been to functions, and someone tells something funny, I'll burst out laughing—and everyone looks at me. The white man has a bit of a grin, a bit of a smile, but that's it. Not me. So we try to reserve our emotion for amongst ourselves; otherwise, we're treated as an oddity.

*How did you meet?*
Heather: We met in the city, as part of a group of Aboriginal and white Christians who had got together to assist the Aboriginal race. I was talking about assimilation, and here was this gentleman sitting across the table from me who flew at me, and said that integration not assimilation was the word. I was absolutely askanced. I thought, 'Who is this man, trying to tell me, a white woman?' And that was Neville Bonner.

Neville: She's learned so much since then through the women folk, and become one of the greatest supporters for the Aboriginal cause that I know. I don't just say that because I love her so much.

*Heather, were you conscious at that first meeting of feeling different?*
Yes, I really think I was. If I look back, I must have felt superior. Could I just put on record the fact that marrying into the Aboriginal culture—and that's what I've done, Neville hasn't married into mine—has been the most rewarding experience of my life, because I have learned so much about living. I have always felt that, when I married Neville, the Aboriginal people stepped over and said, 'Come on in, sister.' They've closed their ranks around me; and I've never known loneliness since, never felt unprotected, because they were always there for me. Mind you, we have had a successful marriage because I did know about Aboriginal culture.

*What have you learned from Neville and the Aboriginal culture?*
The first thing I learned is to never take oneself seriously. The Aboriginal race has such a delightful simple humour. For instance, if you happen to fall down, you're going to be laughed at; so you get yourself up and you laugh. I've also learned to have patience, because I've never yet known a race of people who have such incredible patience. The fact

that we could have taken what—204 years—even to recognise that Aboriginals lived in Australia before we arrived. Yet Aboriginal people patiently waited.

Neville: I think I must intervene here. We were patient for the past 170 years, but in the last twenty-five years or so the younger generation have become darned impatient, and rightly so. They've said to me, 'If we continue to be patient like you or your parents or your grandparents, we will not get anywhere. We want action.' And so they've come out with their protest marches, and they're becoming more articulate, more highly educated. I have never criticised nor condemned the impatient young of my race; because whilst they are doing it in a way that I would not, they are going to get action more quickly than we did by waiting.

*Going back to your relationship between you and your wife, what did you learn from Heather?*

Neville: How much time do we have! I think I've learned that you don't judge people by their colour or their nationality. You judge people from themselves as human beings. Heather has taught me to be more patient, to be more considerate, to think before I open my big mouth too wide, and a whole lot of things along that line. I'm not a formally educated person, whereas my wife has had a high education. Put her education together with my experience and wisdom I have gathered over the years, I often say, 'My love, we're a pretty good team.'

*In the years you have been married, have you been aware of getting older together?*

Heather: Yes we have, and both of us are very philosophical about it. We realise that no matter what age we are in life, we have thoroughly enjoyed it. I'd like to say this to people: Neville is seventy-one, I'll be seventy in a couple of months time, and it's a wonderful age. This is the top of the mountain. You look down and watch other people and think, 'Oh no, I'm glad I'm not struggling up any more.' You know so much, and you've got time—Neville doesn't—time to read wonderful books, and potter in the garden, to watch the grandchildren and the great grandchildren ... things I've looked forward to.

We've both decided, forget about the body. Of course, it's going to have aches and pains (mind you, you have aches and pains when you're younger, too). But it's keeping the mind alive that's important, and respecting youth and their points of view. But oh, wouldn't you agree, darling, that this is a wonderful age to be?

Neville: I am seventy-one, and people say to me, 'What's it like to be seventy-one?' I don't know, haven't got a clue, I'm just Neville. I can't do the things I used to be able to do. One time, if I was going up to Harrods I could walk there in five minutes; now it would probably take me fifteen [the Bonners were in London when they were intereviewed]. I just walk along more casually. There are other things that I can't do, but that doesn't worry me.

When I look back in my youth, I did things in the eyes of my parents and grandparents which were just as bad as the kids are doing today. So I learn to be much more tolerant of young people. They live in a different era to which I lived in. I tried to set standards for my children that were set for me by my parents, and they bucked like heck and went off and did their own thing. But now they're parents and grandparents, they're setting the standards that I was setting for them—one of the most hopeful and heartening things I've seen.

So don't despair of what the young people are doing today; but maintain your standards, because they're going to come back to them. Anyway, let's face it, what has our generation given to them: the atomic bomb, nuclear war, the environment that is now in such disarray? And yet we say, 'Why are they kicking us?' Of course they are, so we must start talking with them and really hear what they say. And then examine why are they saying it, because they are the future of the world. Unless we give them some hope for that future, there is no hope for any of us.

*Do you feel hope?*

Neville: Yes I do. I can't put it into words why I believe that, but I do. I've seen the changes that have occurred within my own situation and my own people. There is light at the end of the tunnel now, and I think I could say this for the rest of the community.

Heather: The thing that really concerns me and I cannot bear it, is the suffering of the children. Do you know Elizabeth Barrett Browning's lines, 'Do ye hear the children weeping, O my brothers ... They are weeping bitterly! They are weeping in the playtime of the others.'? I do hear the children weeping, and I bring it to God's attention all the time. It's the brutality to children that blows me away.

do hear the children weeping, and I bring it to God's attention all the time. It's the brutality to children that blows me away.

*When you talk about God, that seems to be a very strong part of both your lives. Do you share the same beliefs?*

Heather: Yes, we do. I have a very deep Presbyterian belief, and Neville is old-time Baptist; but along with that old-time Baptist is the Aboriginal spirituality. Neville is what I call an old-time Aborigine. Bearing in mind that this gentleman who was a senator for twelve years is only two generations away from the tribe, I think that is quite wonderful. His grandfather was the last initiated member of the Jagera tribe, in whose tribal country we now live—Ipswich and Brisbane. Neville is the last Elder. So he has a lot of these tribal beliefs, and they work.

At first, they were very eerie to me. Neville can get up in the morning and say, 'Oh, number two son will ring today.' So, okay, number two son rings, and I say, 'Oh, hello darling; dad said you would ring.' There are also birds and different things that bring death messages. Whenever I hear the plovers in the park near our home, I think, 'Oh, please don't fly over ours.' I shall never forget when Neville's younger brother was dying from cancer—we cannot mention his name because he is dead. Neville sat by his bed one day and said, 'Brother, the plovers, I've heard the plovers call out.' And that was Neville's way of telling his brother that he was dying. He'd said to the doctor, 'No, don't you tell him; I will tell him when the time is right, through the plover bird.'

We are stupid, Anne; we are stiff upper lip, back to the wall. We are the ones who end up with ulcers. Aborigines grieve. And, of course, if it's a family member or a Jagera member, Neville sings the burial song and, oh, it's pretty primeval, it's magnificent, and all the emotion is let out. I am a great respecter of Aboriginal emotions—instant like a summer storm, then gone. Wonderful! Wouldn't you agree, darling?

Neville: I suppose it's related to Christian faith and our Dreamtime. If you are a Christian, you mourn, and then say you are happy, because your sister or brother, uncle or aunt is now home with Jesus. We say he's gone now, he's in the happy hunting ground with the tribes that have gone on before. So that you grieve at the time because of the loss; but once that's all done, you come to the realisation there's no need to be sorry any more. The spirits are there all the time.

I can walk into my tribal land out in the bush, I can be down in the they're dead.' But the word 'dead' doesn't enter into our vocabulary. They're there in the Dreamtime. The Dreamtime is the beginning, the now, and the after—three things rolled into one. Quite simply, you've got nothing to worry about.

*So how does that affect your attitude about death?*

Neville: As a Christian, the greatest fear I have in my life is that when I go to the happy Dreamtime our God is going to look at me and say, 'Sorry I don't know you. Depart from me.' Well, then I'm going to the unhappy ground, not the happy one. That's the only fear I have. Way back when I was a little boy, grandfather used to say, 'I mightn't know, but He know, He know. You do wrong, I mightn't see you.' So that's part of my living—that some day I've got to pay my rent.

*Heather, what about your attitudes towards death?*

I do agree with Neville. My greatest fear is that I'm not in God's will. So I pray, 'God please keep me in your will.'

*Do you worry about death at all?*

No, not at all. How sad that some people do.

*Do you ever worry about the change in your physical appearance as you grow older?*

No, never. I always say to Neville, 'It costs more and it takes longer.' Again, Anne, you can't have it both ways. You can't have a heap of little great grandchildren and still look forty or fifty, now really! And so the joy is the great grandchildren. I realise that there are some elderly people who do not have great grandchildren, but I do. So that's the way I look at it.

*And do you both take extra care of your health?*

Neville: Heather takes good care of my health, makes sure I eat the right food and have the right amount of rest, once she can nail me down to having a rest. Look, I've been using this body for fifty, sixty years; any damage that was going to be done has already been done.

Heather: Yes, I agree, but I make sure that Neville's blood pressure is checked constantly. I make sure the cholesterol is taken care of, and I make sure we eat all the right vegetables. Neville is absolutely addicted to golf, so he gets the exercise. The doctor has allowed us to smoke because we're watching everything else so terribly, terribly much.

*What have been the elements for you of a happy marriage?*

Heather: You know, I'm terribly old-fashioned, apart from being a Presbyterian and an absolute non-drinker—though I do leave other people to drink because I mind my own business on that—but I believe that in a good marriage a wife must be a wife. I don't mean to be totally subservient, but I really feel not enough women are being wives. I have always kept in the background: been the wife, the secretary, the nursemaid, been the everything. I don't feel that every woman should do that if she doesn't desire; but in our marriage it has worked, by my placating my darling, making sure the house is empty when he comes home—because he's out there in an alien culture all the time.

He says the sweetest music he ever hears is when he comes home and starts to walk up the back steps, and I say, 'Is that you darling?' Of course, I know it's him. And straight away I start to put on the tea kettle and make him a nice strong cup of tea, and we have nice light chitty chat. I realise not everybody can do that, because a big percent of wives nowadays have to work. I haven't had to. Indeed, being the wife of a federal parliamentarian can also be work, because you're the second secretary, the home secretary; you're this, you're that, you can become quite tired in being all dressed up and going out in public. I have put my husband first all the time. I knew it would have to be that way, and I was quite happy to do that. For us it has worked.

*Looking ahead to the next part of your life, are there things you still want to do?*

Heather: [laughs] I'll be very grateful to God if, until I'm called home, we could just go on the way we are, because there are adult grandchildren now who I'm enjoying very much, and then the great grandchildren, and of course our children, too. Gardening, reading all our books, being there for Neville when he comes home from all his wanderings—because he seems to travel so much. No, Anne, just being home with a lovely pussy cat; all these general things one does.

Neville: I think I would just like to play the cards as they fall. I would like to be there if I'm needed, when I'm needed, where I'm needed. There are still a few things that need to be done as far as my own race is concerned and our struggles. But otherwise I just want to stroll down to the barn at my own pace.

*When you die, how would you like to be remembered?*

Neville: Oh dear, as a good father—first should I say a good husband, a good father, and that people will remember the things I've done.

Heather: If you could put on my tombstone, but of course you couldn't [laughs], I would like to have: 'She fought the fight for the Aboriginal race.' I'm worse than Neville. I get up on soap boxes so much more readily, because Neville has been an Aborigine all his life, and he is accustomed to insults. I'm not. I think sometimes I become quite boring, but my whole consuming desire is the fight for the Aboriginal race. And that's what I would like to see on Neville's tombstone: he fought the fight for the Aboriginal race. Because that's what our lives are all about.

Neville: In a sense, I disagree in this respect: whilst I have tried to the best of my ability in the Aboriginal field, I've also tried in my political career to serve all people. So I don't want to be remembered just for one thing. I want to be remembered as a person who has made a contribution to the betterment of my country and my people.

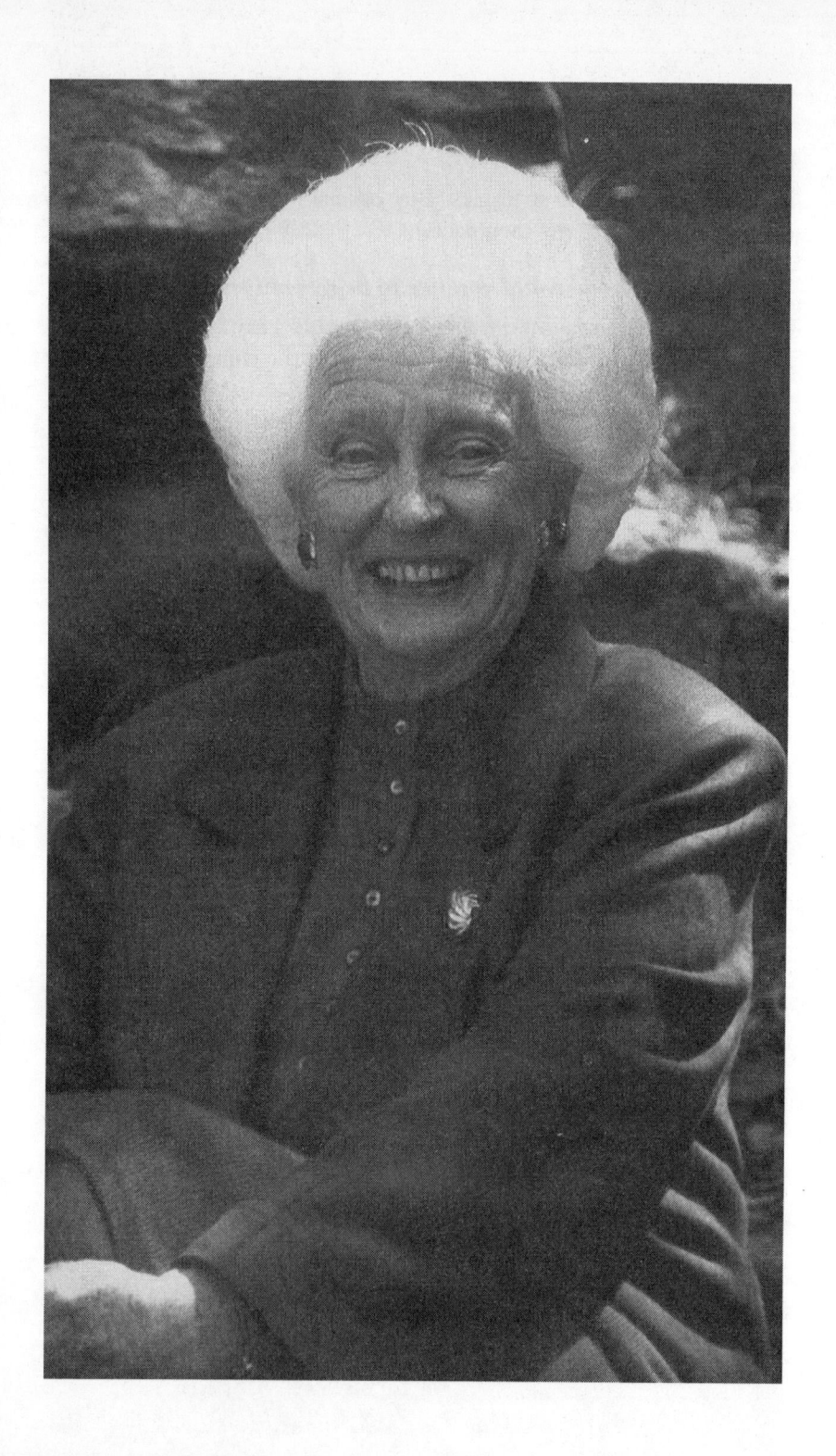

# Beryl Evans
## *I'm going to be a naughty old girl at ninety*

The Honourable Beryl Evans, farmer, grazier, member of the NSW Legislative Council, the premier's official representative on matters affecting older people in New South Wales, was born and spent most of her childhood in Sydney, went into the airforce during the war—almost straight from school—and reached the rank of Section Officer. She still talks about the skills that women acquired during this period, only to lose them when the war ended and they returned to home and family.

She was married in 1944 to a grazier from Dunedoo, and lived there for thirty-two years until her divorce and remarriage in 1976. Beryl Evans was first asked to stand for parliamentary nomination over forty years ago, but decided that her two children (sons) were too young for her to accept the proposal. She remained involved in politics behind the scenes, took a Bachelor of Economics degree at the University of New England in 1981, and was elected to the Senate in 1984. She was given the shadow portfolio of health, and became increasingly interested in the subject of ageing.

Beryl Evans' mother lived until she was two weeks short of ninety, and was a spirited woman full of life. She says that, as a child, her role-models were aunts, mothers, sisters.

All the women I grew up with were very much women of the home—CWAs and flower shows. I remember one of the aunts whose husband had an orchard in Orange: when he died, she'd never even written a cheque. I was born in Sydney at Rockdale, but we moved house a lot because my younger brother had very bad asthma, and there was always the theory that he might be better in the mountains. When that didn't work, we'd come back into the city areas. So I went to quite a few schools over time. I finished up at MLC in Burwood. My father was in the motor business. All the family were in the motor business. I was married in 1944 when I was still in the airforce, and stayed in till the end of 1945, and then went back to the country as I had married a country fellow. I lived there for thirty-two years, just outside Dunedoo.

*Was ageing something you ever thought about?*

No, I don't think so. I can remember thinking when the kids were little, 'What would happen to my children if I died young?' But other than that ... Anne, I heard someone say the other day, 'I don't feel any different.' And you *don't* feel any different, but it's only your body that doesn't do what it's supposed to do, or stay the way it's supposed to stay. It's terribly important to be doing things, to keep your mind active and alert. I think that's what keeps you young, if that is possible.

*Have changes in your physical appearance worried you?*

I often look at myself in the morning and think, 'My God, what's happened to me!' But I would never have a face lift or things like that, and I've never dyed my hair. I think nature's kind to you the way it helps soften what's there. There are times when I am tired and I can see my mother—it's just amazing— so I think that's how I'll look when I'm ninety. It worries me that I'm not keeping as fit as I should. I used to be very keen about jogging and all sorts of things, but now I just don't get time. I'd like to be fitter than I am. I play golf and tennis when I can, and I've started on an exercise campaign this week to try and get ready for the summer. I swim in the summer; I think that's great.

*Do you find you get more tired?*

No, I have moments of being tired. I'm a great vitamin-taker. I think Lady Cilento was very wise with her vitamin theories, and my doctor tells me I'm a good example of what vitamins can do. I'm very good at picking up. I can go and lie down and sleep for fifteen minutes, and get up and go again. But I think you're made that way: you've either got that kind of vitality, or you haven't.

*Do you think you're wiser now?*
I know a lot more, but whether I use it in the right way I don't know. I find I'm intolerant at times. I get cross with the wheel being reinvented over and over again. I think you're always learning. I've got the wonderful experience of being elected here by both houses of parliament onto the executive of this Commonwealth Parliamentary Association. And when you ask, 'How are women going in the world?,' in an executive of twenty-four, I'm the only woman out of fifty nations—which is amazing, isn't it. That's made me a jet-setter. Out of the blue, I'm whizzing off all over the place. It's fascinating the women I'm meeting from all over the world.

*Do you think that people treat you differently because you are a woman and an older woman?*
They've suddenly realised how old I am, and that's an enigma to them [laughs]. Yes, they really don't quite know what to do with me, because I cover the ground faster than most of them and get more things done, and that infuriates them. And they don't think I should be here. If you heard what the Premier said the other day—that he now has a 'young energetic cabinet'! I think that's amazing, that youth is the goal all the time.

*When you read something like that, how does it affect you?*
It's immature, because with the parliaments that I am mixing with now, Australia seems to be the only country that has this lure of the young. Most of the politicians from India and Africa and other countries are all middle aged or more.

*I wonder why that is?*
Hasn't Australia always been the country of sunburnt, golden young people? We have been a young nation, but with the changing numbers, that's where governments have got to take another look at things. There's going to be two million people over the age of sixty-five by the year 2000. America will have a million people over one hundred years

of age. It just makes your mind boggle. And the majority of those are well. They're not sick. As I tell everyone when I go out, we used to say, 'Well dear old thing, you've turned sixty; sit down there and be a good girl, and we'll forget about you.' That's not happening any more. They're up and doing, getting out and helping people, and they're being counted. Governments have got to realise that. And, of course, the more they do, the better it is. The cost of sick people is enormous.

*Looking back, what was the life of old people like?*
When I first came into parliament I used to see lots of sick old people who just seemed to sit in chairs and do nothing. That upset me terribly, and in the country particularly they seemed to be just sitting and knitting. They'd never go out at night, for instance. The CWAs and the Red Cross with their afternoon meetings, that was the only time they went out. There was no incentive to try things or do things. When I opened a conference in Chatswood last year, and I went round talking to some of them, one lady was beautifully dressed and very excited, and I said, 'Tell me what you're doing.' And she said, 'I've learned to paint. Isn't that fabulous!' I said, 'How old are you?', and she said, 'Eighty-five.' She never knew she could do it before, and now has a new world for herself. Another group said, 'Look, we all meet here, and once a month we go out—we don't care where—we might get on a train and go as far as it'll go. We go to meet new people.' They're *living* instead of just sitting at home. And because we live longer than the men it's very difficult for a woman who's just been a housewife and a mother and done the normal sort of things, when a husband dies, to come out alone and make that break.

*Does that take a lot of courage?*
Tremendous courage, but I think that's what these groups are doing now. You know the 'RSVP' which I'm fascinated with? It's the Retired Seniors' Volunteers Program. They go to people and say, 'Would you like to do something voluntary, some work?' I found, for instance, some elderly men planting trees, and then they're getting teachers who've retired going back to school to help kids who are having reading problems. They've got the time and patience to do it, and they're mixing again with kids—which they love doing. That's fantastic, because it's a completely new life for them instead of just playing bowls or sitting at home watching TV.

*It's interesting how we do put limitations on people, particularly old people. What are some of the most common limitations you've come across?*

I think health. The person who's become old and just sits, gives up, I think. And so many are overweight, so it's an effort to move about anyway. And of course children have become a problem, because they think it's wrong for mum to be out doing all those sort of things. I'm lucky, because my sons have always said, 'For God's sake, get up and do it; there's no reason why you can't.' I went back and did an economics degree as an external student at New England University and graduated in 1981, because my elder son said it was time I did something constructive. It was jolly hard, but it was great to go back and mix with all those people and go into residence and find yourself a student. I loved it.

*Do you think that attitudes towards men when they get older, are different from attitudes towards women?*

Yes. I think they are inclined to say, 'Isn't he wonderful—he's still driving his car, and he's still playing his bowls, and he's still got his meetings.' They're always surprised when women are doing things, very surprised. The actress, Colleen Clifford, she's ninety-six, I think: I took her out to Westmead Hospital and we both launched a health kit together. She's quite out of this world. She lives in a lovely old terrace in Sydney with two actors who look after her. She says, 'Just bring me cups of tea, dear, nothing else,' and they tell me that she rarely gets in before three in the morning. When I drove her back she wanted to get out at St Mary's Cathedral to go to one o'clock Mass. She got out of the car, and waved as she went. She has trouble with her legs, but she doesn't let that defeat her.

*Is there a tendency to talk about older people and to older people as if they were stupid?*

If you are in hospital, that's how they treat you anyway. They'll discuss you outside the door as if you can't hear. And I suppose they do do that in these nursing homes—they treat them as children. They say they're in their second childhood; that's what they keep telling them all the time—which is a tragedy, because there are things these people can do. The main thing is to get them moving. It breaks my heart to just see them staring into space. I know there's not much they want to do, perhaps, but I think this idea now of bringing in animals is wonderful. When I visited a retirement home in Cobar recently, outside each person's door is a photograph of themselves and in the hall is a lovely big basket for the dog, and the dog's photograph. The interest they take in that dog! They want to take him for a walk, whereas they wouldn't walk for the nurse.

*When you married for a second time was there a reaction to this?*
It was a great shock to have been married for thirty-two years and then get a divorce. Some of my friends were shocked; others said we were the only ones that had enough sense to do it. It's not an easy thing to do. Luckily, on my side of it, my first husband and I are good friends; he lives on the property with my younger son, and I go and visit him, and he comes and visits us. I find I get both husbands ganging up on me occasionally, which isn't a very good experience. But my present husband had a very difficult time with his divorce; it wasn't a pleasant experience at all.

*I was thinking about the actual ritual of getting married, because in the past there was an expectation that over a certain age you just didn't remarry.*
Oh, I was swept off my feet more than I've ever been swept off in my life. There is still romance if you love someone.

*But is there is still an assumption that people don't fall in love over a certain age, that it's not even quite seemly?*
Yes. Isn't it incredible? The young can do anything they like, but the older ones aren't supposed to. But when you see a marriage of a really old couple, everyone's shocked and horrified. I think that's nonsense. There's always love in people. I love the story of the man whose wife died, and the family became very worried about him and decided the only thing to do was put him in a retirement village. He was absolutely furious, but they moved the poor old fellow in; and so he refused to see the family.

About six months later he rang his daughter and invited her to lunch. She was delighted. She went to see him, and they were talking about everything, when he suddenly said to her, 'Are diamonds very expensive today?' When she'd got her breath back, he confessed that he'd fallen in love with one of the ladies of the place and they were going to get engaged. I think it happens more than people realise, but there's not a great deal of publicity because of what you say—it's not expected of older people, and people think it's not on.

*And people actually used to be segregated, even husbands and wives.*
Yes, because of what's just been said. They said the same thing about paraplegic people, who nowadays get married and have children; and nobody thinks that's odd any more. But once they would have been isolated and thought indecent if they fell in love again. Oh no, I hope that never stops. I've always told them I'm going to be a naughty old girl at ninety, because I've never been game to be naughty at other times.

*Have you found that with age comes a certain kind of liberation?*
No, I think I've always enjoyed living. I learned very early in life that you can plan ahead to a certain extent, but you just do not know what's round the corner. I'm very much for enjoying today and then see what comes tomorrow.

*Do you have any particular religious beliefs?*
I believe in God very much, yes. I've had great support from that. I'm not a great church-goer by any means, but my second son had polio when he was only five, before the vaccine, and my father had cancer very badly. I think when you go through things like that you get a faith. None of my family has been good church-goers, but there's always been a very real belief. I find that a great comfort.

*Do you think that, when you die, the essence of you continues?*
Oh, that's a big question. I don't know, I really don't. I think we like to believe that there's something there. There are times when you wonder why you do things as if you are being guided. Sometimes that makes you think.

*You were talking about your feeling that you hadn't changed; that deep inside you were the same as when you were little.*
Always an extrovert, always! I can remember writing plays at school, and getting all the kids to do them and dressing up, always busy doing something. I remember mummy telling me that a cook we had called me Miss Affectation Demonstration.

*When we look back at our lives we sometimes measure them in peaks and troughs. What were some of yours?*

I think my experience in the Air Force was just a tremendous thing. I was only sad that there had to be a war to do that, because being an only daughter and a very protected little girl to go into that field was a wonderful experience for me. I started as an ACW, the lowest rank, and trained as a drill instructor and a PT instructor, and then was commissioned. Having my children: I love my sons very dearly and they still are a wonderful joy. Being married both times. Coming in here, and the committee that I'm on now: I didn't expect anything like that to happen towards the end of my career. My grandchildren, that's another peak: they're great. The troughs have been ... well, my son Gawain's illness—the disability that he's gained from that has always been a terrible blow; my mother and father—I think I've missed them terribly. I had a great relationship with my father and my mother. They were always wonderful to go and talk to.

*If you think of the kind of things that are available now to old people, is there still a long way to go?*

Oh yes, there are still tremendous hurdles; and, Anne, the problem is that when we talk about older people, we've got a generation out there now, the forties and over, who are out of work, and they will probably never go out into the workforce again. They're not old, but there's got to be things for them to do and things to keep them going. They're an absolute tragedy, because they've got young families and mortgages, and they must be absolutely desperate out there. We are going to have tremendous problems. Those people are going to live a long time, and the numbers frighten me a bit. It's good for everybody to be doing things, but just how many things are there to do?

I would love to see the older people being used more than they are by youth itself. I know you can't put an old head on young shoulders, but experience is good, and if you mix them all together you get something better. I was thrilled by all these older retired people going back into the schools, because there's nothing better than when a little kid falls over and is in tears, and a grey haired granny can pick them up; whereas a teacher hasn't got time to do that. And, strangely enough I think kids love to talk to older people, just somebody who will sit and listen, because professionals do the most wonderful job, but they are bound to professional duties, aren't they? The dedication of people who do these things is just incredible. I've been out to Prince Henry to see some of the people working with AIDS in the palliative centre, and you know those nurses! I spoke to one of them and I said, 'How do you face up to it, day after day?' And she said, 'Well, you feel sometimes you've achieved things; you've helped.' I find that dedication is just incredible. The fear of dying and helping people to die is something that's just got to be looked at.

*Do you think about dying yourself?*
Not very often, but sometimes I do.

*Does that worry you?*
No, not really. I know it's got to come. I'm going to be disappointed. There are a lot of things I'd like to do. Sometimes, you think you'd like to go on living for ever.

*What are some of the things you'd like to do?*
Oh well, a lot more travel, and a number of places I'd love to go to. I'd like to see my grandchildren have children. I think that would be wonderful, to see what they are like. I'd like to do a lot more sport than I do. I love skiing—but then I'm not a good skier—and I'd love to go back and live on the snow for six months and really ski well again.

*Do you worry about hurting yourself? It doesn't sound as if you do.*
I sometimes worry on the road, because I realise that you're tempting fate when you travel as much as I do. The accidents and the driving are terrifying. There are times when you have near misses and you think, 'Golly me, that would be terrible.' But otherwise, I climb up ladders and paint ceilings, jump around all over the place. I don't think I really worry about hurting myself, no.

*How would you like to be remembered?*
As a person who enjoyed life, who loved people and this wonderful land. A lover of animals and birds, big and small. And a warm, kind person who helped other people.

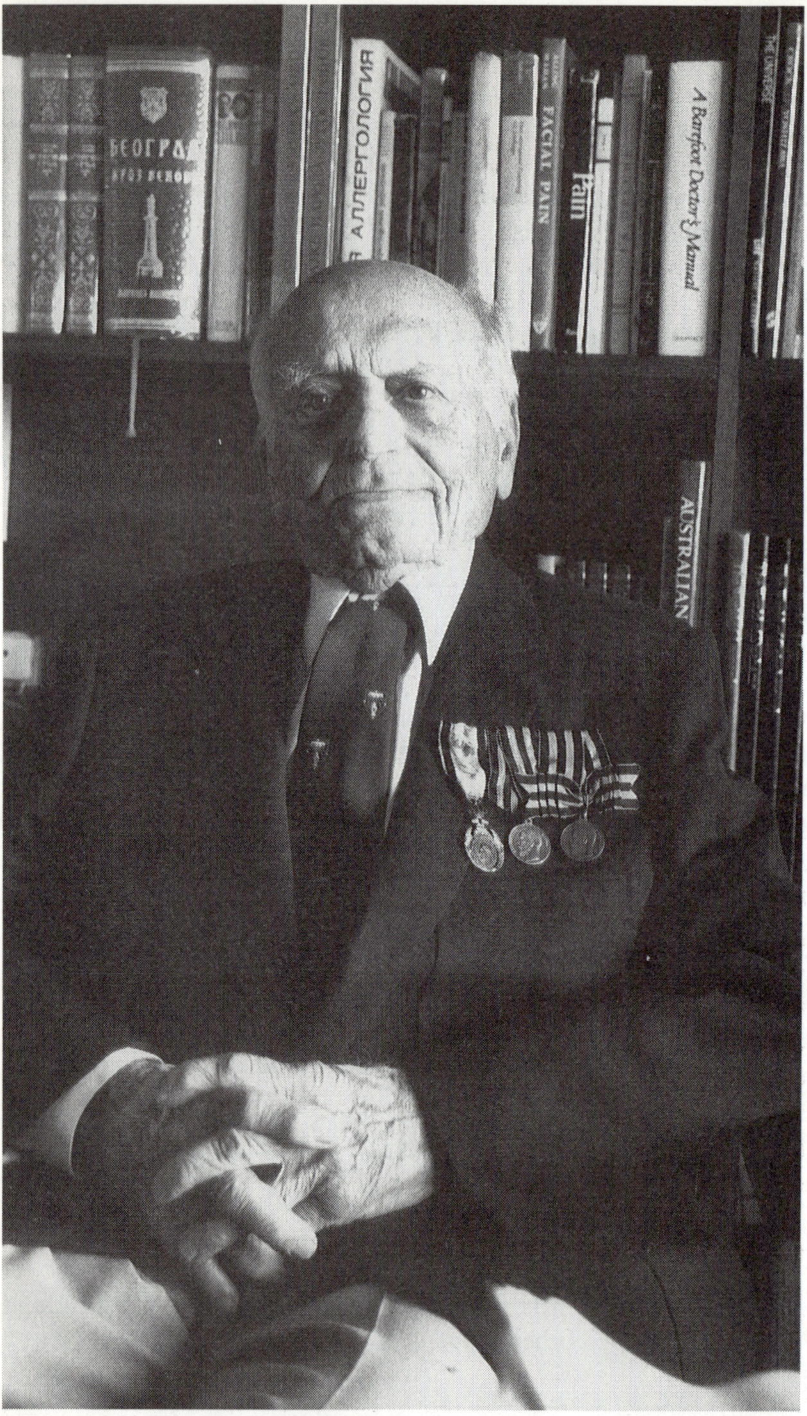
АЛЛЕРГОЛОГИЯ
FACIAL PAIN
Pain
A Barefoot Doctor's Manual
AUSTRALIAN

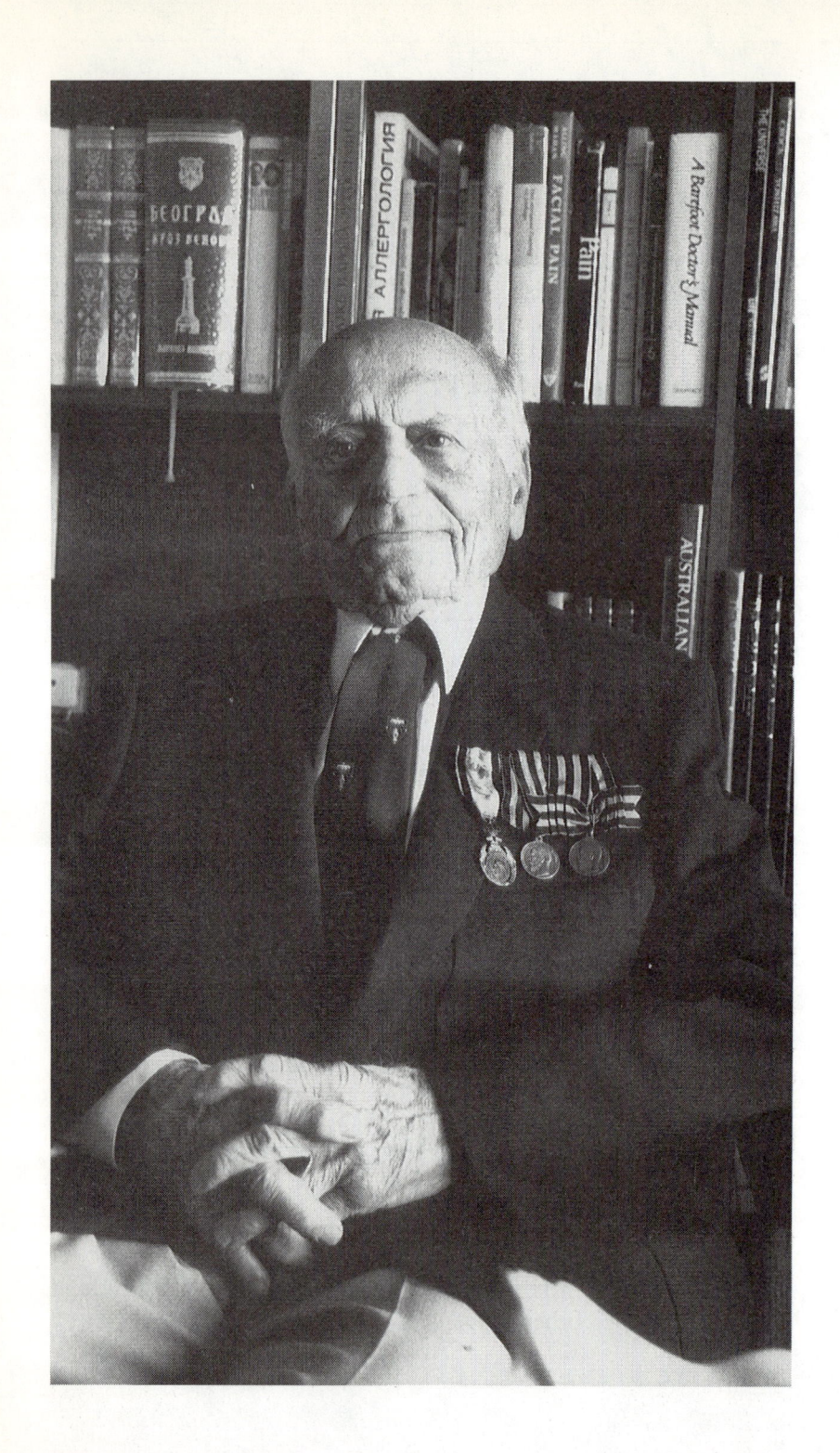

# Bogdan Stojic
*I'm 101. I will stop work*

Dr Bogdan Stojic was still practising medicine when he was one hundred years old. One year later, in 1994, he decided it was time to give up. Now he reads, writes, goes for walks, and enjoys his many friends.

He was born in Croatia—then part of the Austro-Hungarian empire—in 1893, the year that Henry Ford built his first motor car, Toulouse Lautrec was painting at the Moulin Rouge, and Gladstone was prime minister of Great Britain. In 1911, when Stojic was eighteen, he enrolled in the faculty of medicine in Graz, Austria and qualified in Vienna nine years later. He says it took him this length of time because between 1912 and 1918 he had to fight in three wars: the Balkan war against Turkey, the Serbo-Bulgarian war, and World War One. In World War Two, he was a surgeon in five prisoner-of-war camps along with Russian, French, British, and Australian and New Zealand soldiers. He has worn the uniform of seven armies, received two medals for bravery, and twice been sentenced to death by firing squad. After World War Two ended, he worked in a Zagreb hospital as a surgeon, before setting up his own private practice in sclerotherapy and later in neural therapy.

He migrated to Australia with his wife Marusa in 1965, to join their daughter Irina. His daughter says that he taught her Russian and English, how to brush her teeth properly, how to blow her nose, and how to dance the Russian men's dance 'Kazatchok'.

My parents were ninety, but I never thought about it—how old I live. It just happened. I will not say it is a shock. Why did it happen? I tell you this, I was prisoner of war in Germany, and I saw for one year every day at seven o'clock in the morning a big wagon, maybe with fifty carcasses of horses, who were at least six or seven days dead. And I ate for one year these dead carcasses; for one year, because otherwise I couldn't live! So when the patients ask me, 'How is it that you have reached such an old age?' I tell them this. But it is a joke [chuckles].

*Do you think that people can lengthen their lives?*
Yes. If they don't smoke and don't drink too much.

*Do you smoke or drink?*
Never. Only one day in my life. I was ten years of age and I saw my uncle, he was smoking, and I took a cigarette. I tried it, and I started to vomit. I said, 'Never more, never more.' That's my luck, I've always said so.

*It's been my luck, too. I have no tolerance for it. Do you think we will be able to prolong human life?*
Yes, by telling them: don't smoke; don't drink too much. And also don't take such dangerous sports like football. I have seen broken necks from the scrummage.

*Are there advantages in being old?*
There are many younger people who are my friends, and they visit to speak with me.

*And disadvantages?*
Yes. If you are sick. I am worrying with the sick, because of my discs. All the lumbar and three in the neck, they are old. But there is a doctor who will give me injections, and I got such injections into the nerve on the spinal canal, and I was improved.

*What sort of a doctor are you?*
I have been a surgeon, phlebologist, and neural therapist. As a phlebologist, I treated varicose veins and haemorrhoids. Neural therapy, that's treatment of different diseases using local anaesthetic injections.

There is a book about neural therapy; it includes 393 different diseases which are treated with one injection.

*How important is the relationship between the doctor and the patient in healing someone?*
If the patient believes he or she will be cured, that is very important. Otherwise, he will not come. There are very seldom patients who will come once and then not again. That's the exception.

*Going back in your life, you have been in several wars; can you tell me about them?*
The first war was against Turkey in 1912. The Serbs were five hundred years under the Turkish rule, and many of them changed religion, became Muslims, to have a better chance in life. You hear every day about Muslims from Bosnia Herzegovena. They are mostly Serbs and some Croats. You can change the political approach, but you can't change your nationality. But, in 1970, Tito proclaimed the Serb and Croat Muslims only Muslims.

*Do you think anything is ever achieved by war?*
By this war, no. This is not war.

*But you have fought in wars?*
Yes. I was mobilised in Austria, in the Austrian army. The Serbs kicked out the Austrian army three times, so as a Serb I tried to escape. I was a medical student. I had five soldiers with me, and always three or four hundred metres behind the front line. This is very dangerous. When I escaped I started to cry. I couldn't stop, and they asked me, 'Tell us, maybe they have killed your family?' 'No, I am crying because I am having luck, and being happy because I am among you.'

I said, 'I would like to benefit you. I would like to remain with you and fight with you.' 'No,' they said. 'We can't do it here on the front line, you must go and talk to the commander of the army.' So I came to the commander, and he persuaded me that as a medical student I am more valuable than a fighter. I said to them, 'You are right' [laughs]. I remained working in the hospital, and my chief was a Russian professor from Siberia. A very good surgeon. I was his assistant and then, when the Germans came to aid the Austro-Hungarian army, they attacked with great force and we retreated through Albania. I had not changed my shirt; it was on my body for six weeks. You can imagine what I looked like! When we retreated, it was the command of the government that all boys from twelve to sixteen should be taken with the army. Many thousands of these youngsters died or were slaughtered by Albanians.

*Why do you think we show such brutality to each other?*

Because people have such twisted brains with religion, with politics, with argument. Nobody can change my beliefs. I have friends of all kinds of peoples of different nations here, particularly here. And I have never felt to be enemy to Chinese, to Aborigines, to Jews. I have very great friends—Jews—and I was very disturbed when I heard Hitler had killed six million Jews. Six million.

*Did you at any stage nearly die in those wars?*

Oh yes, I was sentenced to death. In Germany, by the German Gestapo; and by the Jugoslav communists immediately upon my return home when the war ended. The Gestapo leader—a Baron—he came to our camp where the prisoners were. They were all intelligent: priests, schoolteachers, engineers.

One day, the German doctor who was in the camp for the prisoners of war—a very nice man—saw me and asked me to put the French men who were sick on a list. When the French Vichy government agreed to collaborate with Hitler, the German government allowed all French prisoners who were sick to be repatriated. I asked the French prisoners to put down their symptoms, and said I would give it to the German doctor, and he would recommend that they would be repatriated. I put two hundred and fifty on the list, and with the first train they were sent to France. Two hundred and fifty men: this was for me such a joy!

But then came the Gestapo: he had heard about this, and he went down to the commandant of the whole camp, and said, 'Dr Stojic will be executed this moment! Today! Now!' The commandant was a colonel and a very nice man; he was professor at high school, and he said, 'You can't do it. You can't do it here'. They came to me and showed me a booklet saying I was to be killed by firing squad. The commandant escorted me to a place where there was a young girl sitting and using typing machine, and crying and trembling because she had read what was going to happen. But in the end the commandant got my transfer out of there to another camp where there were five thousand Russian prisoners of war. Every day, five hundred new ones came in and five hundred were sent to the cemetery. So I was there for six months. And they waited for me also to die. I did not.

*Were you frightened at the time?*
No, only for the first time when this girl was shivering. I thought, 'They will execute me today.' I was frightened.

*Do you have any religion?*
Yes, Serb Orthodox. I believe there is something which we can't understand what it is here. We must obey.

*Has that grown stronger as you have got older?*
Not really. It was always so.

*Do you believe that there is a purpose for each person's life? Do you believe in any kind of destiny?*
No.

*Do you believe there is any kind of life after we die?*
I am not sure.

*Why did you come to Australia?*
My daughter and her husband were planning to go to Canada or Australia. My son-in-law is a traffic engineer. He came to Zagreb and worked hard for three years as a chief engineer in a big car-repair shop. His boss was a Communist Paty member and my son-in-law wasn't. Also, as a university graduate, my son-in-law was considered unproductive and bourgeois. One day, in an argument, this manager banged his fist on the table and shouted: 'The day will come when we won't need engineers any longer.' My son-in-law decided it was time to leave.

We had two connections to Australia: Dr Norman Rose, superintendent of Sydney Hospital, who had spent the last two years of war with me sharing the same room in the prisoner-of-war camp; and my daughter's school friend, who had settled in Sydney.

*Has Australia been a good place for you?*
Oh, yes. We really like Australia; we feel here better than in Jugoslavia,

much better. Very nice country! But there are so many unemployed. We must stop it. Australia has everything except a glacier, and this can be done. Kosciusko can be raised up 1500 metres and there will be a glacier. If the old Egyptians constructed those pyramids without great machines, why should we not raise Kosciusko?

*Why would we want to?*
We would have a glacier, and we would have a great amount of water. This water you could make for electricity. Many other good things would come from it.

*Have you written about this?*
No, I will [laughs]. All those unemployed can work. There will be plenty of workers.

*Do you have lots of ideas?*
Yes. In medicine, though the doctors will not accept it. I am astonished.

*Do you still read scientific journals; do you keep up to date?*
Yes, I get three journals.

*What is a typical day for you?*
How I spend my day? Reading. First, medical journals and the papers about politics. And then my dictionary, always learning new words.

*Do you walk at all now?*
Yes, but very difficult. I'll be treated. Soon, I hope I will walk without the stick.

*When your short term memory goes, does it irritate you?*
Yes [chuckles], but I can remember things clearly in the past. Many things.

*What have been the most important things to you in your life?*
That I have very good parents. My father and mother were very good. They spoke with us as if we were grown-up people when we were ten years of age.

*And now with your wife and your daughter?*

Yes, my marriage has been very good.

*Where did you meet your wife?*

It was in Zagreb. I was there, and I met her because there was a high percentage of Russians, and I speak Russian. Her father had a big Wienna coffee house in Ljubljana and a restaurant in Zagreb. And so I met her there. She was eighteen years old. She is Sovene.

*What do you think helps make a marriage a good marriage?*

Friends. You must be friends.

*Looking ahead, are there things you would still like to do?*

Yes. I would like to help Alzheimer's with local anaesthetic (zylocaine) injections to the brain. It increases the blood circulation. I am interested in this but, because I have ceased to practise, I can't do it.

*Did you mind giving up your practice? Was that difficult?*

No. I thought, 'I'm 101. I will stop it.'

*How do people treat you now that you are over a hundred? Have they changed their attitude at all?*

Not really. My old patients are sorry that I'm not working any more.

*People can be very patronising toward old people. Do people ever patronise you?*

No, they would not do this to me. All my acquaintances are my good friends, and I have several nationalities as friends; and many Australians, real Australians, very good friends.

*So friendship has been very important in your life?*

Yes, yes, yes.

*How would you like to be remembered?*

As a doctor.

*And for your other qualities, your qualities as a man, how would you like to be remembered?*

I don't know. I think they will have a good memory about me—all my patients and friends.

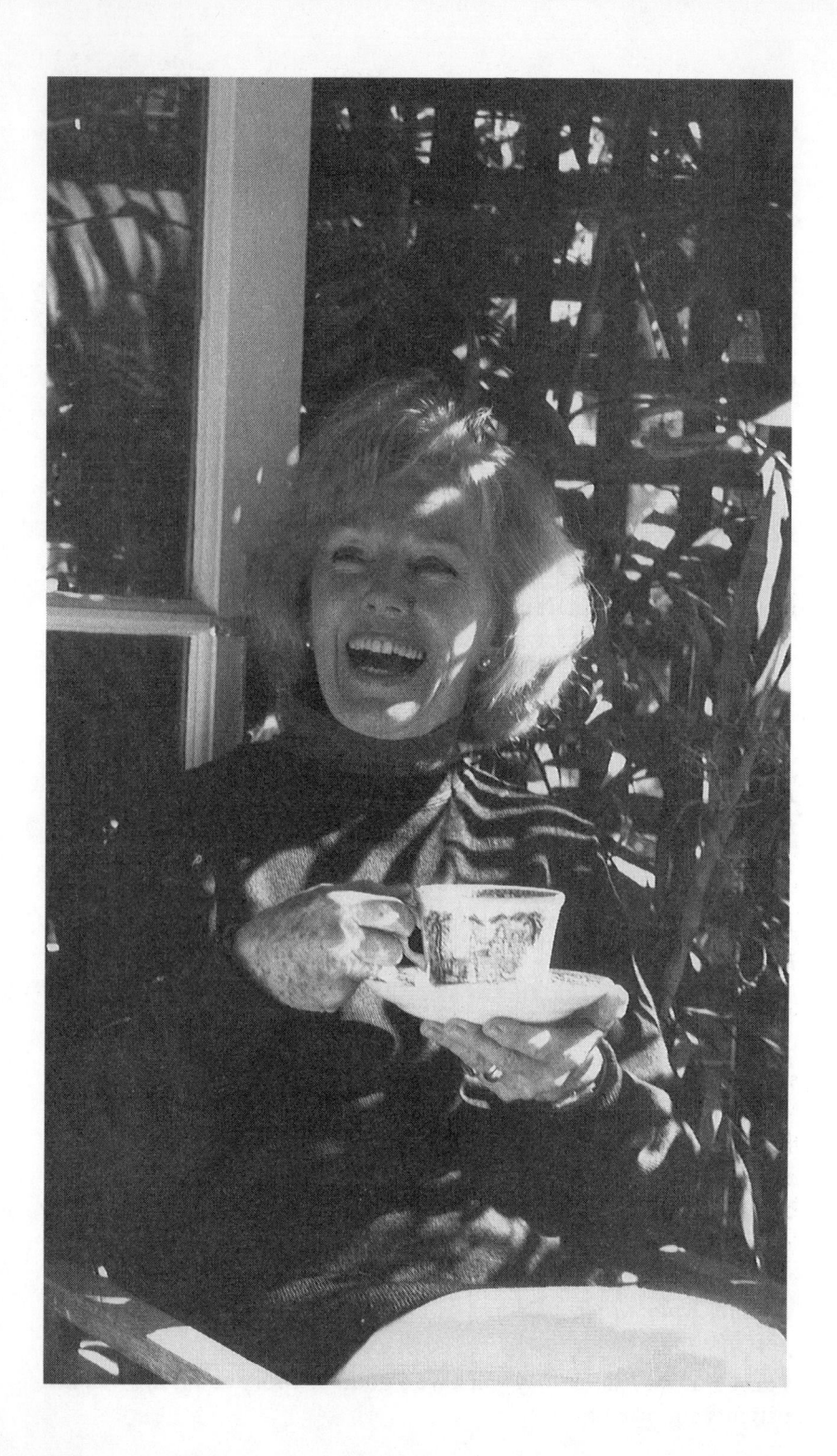

# Carol Raye
*Something our family is used to*

Carol Raye has had a long and very successful career in England, America, and Australia as an actor, dancer, and entertainer. She was born in England, trained as a ballet dancer before several West End successes in musicals, and then put her career on hold when she married Robert Ayre-Smith, a veterinarian and agricultural scientist. They lived first in the United States and then in Kenya on a 10,000-acre experimental farm in the Rift Valley, heart of Mau Mau terrorist activity. She raised funds for local hospitals, and organised the first ever multi-racial women's group in the region. The last three years in Kenya were spent in Nairobi, where she joined the television department of the Kenya Broadcasting Corporation as a producer/director.

She and her husband and their three chilren settled in Australia in 1964, were naturalised, and have lived here ever since. Carol Raye is perhaps best known for her role in Australia's first weekly satirical television program, *The Mavis Brampston Show*, for which she won a Best Actress Logie Award in 1964. She has served on the Theatre Board of the Australia Council, stood for pre-selection as a Liberal Party senator—and nearly won—and now doesn't belong to any political parties. She argues tenaciously with her left-wing friends, and has a strong sense of family.

My grandparents were the most influential older people that I knew. They were in my life for a long time, because they both lived to a ripe old age. My grandmother was a very strong woman. She had to be—she went to work when she was still a child in a family where her father had died. They were very poor, and there were a lot of brothers and sisters.

I remember her saying that she went to a factory to try and get a job, because she could sew. In those days, you didn't get ready-made clothing; all the dresses were hand-made. The foreman said to her, 'How old are you?' She said she was eleven, and he said, 'Spell "work".' She said, "w-o-r-k". Then he said, 'Spell "walk." And when she hesitated, he said, 'Look, come back later, because I think you should do a bit more schooling.' It was such a sweet story, because she was obviously very young.

But she did go back, and she worked very hard all her life. When she married my grandfather, I remember stories of taking in lodgers, because she was determined that she would educate her three children to a much better way of life. And this she achieved. My father went into the navy, and my uncle into the civil service.

My grandmother was more dominant than my grandfather. He was a very tall good-looking man, and I remember him telling me lovely stories. He was a clever carpenter; he could do anything with his hands. He was with the Thames Water Police, and they had these wonderful, extraordinary whistles. I still have my grandfather's whistle, which I keep in my handbag. When my grandparents became very old, they came to live with my parents; and then later my parents lived with me. My cousin has exactly the same philosophy, because she looked after her parents until they died and is very close to her children now. I think this is something that our family is used to.

*What do you remember about your grandmother?*

Oh, because she had been a very fine seamstress she always had wonderful boxes of Victorian buttons, and one of the treats when I was little was to go and look at her button boxes. Out would come these buttons, which now would be very valuable. I don't know what happened to them, these glorious buttons and trimmings, and all sorts of things in her sewing cupboard. I remember being very cold when I was about three or four, and grandmamma warming newspaper in front of the fire and wrapping it round my feet, and saying, 'There's nothing like warm newspaper to warm your feet.'

She had a wonderful gold muff chain, very long, on the end of which she always had her pocket watch; and every dress she wore had a little pocket. When she died, she gave the muff chain to me and the watch to my cousin, and I wear it to this day. She wasn't beautiful, but she had a strong face. She was young in the era when people were nervous of the camera; so in every picture of grandmamma when she was young, she really doesn't look wonderful. She was not tall, about five foot two, whereas my grandfather was about six foot one; but she was slim and upright to the end of her days, and she had lovely white hair which she used to put on the top of her head. She was a beautiful person.

*As she got very old, do you remember any feelings you had about her? Lots of children are frightened of old people because they think they smell strange.*

Well, she always smelled gorgeous, my grandmamma, and I was never frightened of her. Nor of my grandfather, who had very white hair and a moustache—again, very upright. No, they were very protective people in my mind, very special, and I always looked forward to seeing them. My mother's parents, I didn't know at all. Her father died before I was born, and my mother's mother died when I must have been about one or two. So my paternal grandparents were really the only grandparents I had.

*As a child, what were you like?*

I had a lovely life. I was an only child, and in some ways I was spoiled. But even though my parents were not particularly well off, I never had any feelings of wanting things I couldn't have. There always seemed to be something to do. I remember spending hours drawing fashions and making clothes. I had dancing lessons from when I was about four. I had a natural ability, so I enjoyed my dancing lessons. However, because my parents were nothing to do with the theatre, I never thought about doing anything with that ability. I just thought that maybe one day I would be a dancing teacher.

When I was fifteen, a local amateur dramatic society in Portsmouth, where we lived, was going to do a musical called *No, No, Nanette*. The leading role of Nanette had to be somebody much younger than they had in their company, somebody who could sing and dance and look right for the part. It was suggested that I should audition, and I got the role. It was a great success, so then I persuaded my parents to let me leave school, and I went full time to dancing school. I took all my ballet exams from the Royal Academy, and then we heard of a new school being opened in London by Freddie Carpenter, who was a London choreographer and an Australian, and my mother asked him if he would see me. She took me up to London, and I did my little song and dance—mummy played the piano beautifully. I sang a Jessie Mathews song, and wore a brown chiffon dress mummy had made me. And he said, yes, he'd take me in his school.

We never started the classes, because we got a telegram the following week to say he was doing the choreography in a new musical in London with Stanley Lupino and Florence Desmond at Her Majesty's, and he thought the ingenue lead was something I could do. On the dress rehearsal, the young leading lady, Sally Grey, hurt herself in one of the dance routines, and I had to go on for opening night—not even having had an understudy rehearsal. Every London manager was there because it was a big show, so I was then asked to do other shows before I'd even appeared in London. That's how I got into the theatre; all quite by accident. I did about five big musicals in London and about four films, so I had a very good career.

*Has getting older surprised you?*

Oh, I don't know about surprised me. At times it's irritating, when I now realise there are certain things I will never be able to do. For instance, I took up skiing when I must have been about forty. Now I know I will never be a good skier. I know I will never have my face on the front of *Time* magazine. There are limitations as you get old; that's the only boring part. But getting old is quite interesting, because your mind alters and your desires change in tune with your age; you don't regret not going disco dancing any more, because in fact you don't really want to go disco dancing. And you don't wish you had lots of money to buy lots and lots of diamonds, because you don't really want those things any more. I don't bother about clothes like I used to; I dress to be comfortable.

So I don't think getting old surprises me, and I've been blessed—touch wood—with good health. Your viewpoint of growing old depends entirely on your health. If you are crippled with arthritis, your outlook on life is going to be very different.

*Some people talk about being surprised that they are seventy or eighty, because they don't feel that particular age.*

Yes, you feel in your mind exactly the same. The world all looks as it should, and then you suddenly see in a shop window a middle-aged person going past, and realise it is you. I went into the theatre when I was very young, and was always the youngest in everything I did: the youngest in the show, the youngest dancer, the youngest actress. So that when people are deferential in my profession, you suddenly realise that you are the older generation now; but you don't feel any different in yourself.

*Is there anything else you would like to do that you now know you can't? And anything you still want to do that you could?*

I'd love to be able to play the piano like mother did. I would loved to have danced with Fred Astaire, because I was good enough. I was considered one of the top dancers in London in my time, and therefore it's not like a fantasy, and because, like every dancer, one admired him so. I suppose I regret not actually working in the States. I did one top musical there, in which I got very good reviews; and I had the opportunity of staying on in a musical review that became a great hit, but my parents were sick in England, and I felt that I had to go back.

As to things that I could still do, I'd like to learn French and Indonesian. I would like to write—mainly for my children—a record of what I have done. I've got a lot to say about what I think is wrong with things in the world: political things to do with our society, which seems to me to be taking the wrong direction. I firmly believe in small is beautiful, and freedom of choice, and certain ethics where you do as much for yourself as you can, and you only ask the government to help when all else has failed.

It seems to me we're moving more and more into a society where people are taught the government should look after you from cradle to the grave, parents are really irrelevant, and whether you've got two doesn't really matter—one will do—and if one is not very good, come to the social welfare and somebody will pick up the pieces. So all the values I've been brought up with, I see being whittled away. That wouldn't matter if it looked as if people were having a better time than I had. But I don't see that. And therefore I'd like to see some changes in education, and philosophical thinking about society.

*Do you feel that age has brought wisdom?*
[Hilarious laughter] My husband doesn't think so. I remember Robert saying to me once, 'I thought that as you grew older you would have grown wiser.' I think I have. I don't know if it's self-evident. I think you do learn to be less selfish as you get older, and you realise there are other people around you. The people around you have points of view that don't necessarily coincide with yours. And you learn to count to ten. I'm Irish, you see, and the Irish in me is quite volatile; so that I'm apt to go in hard when I sometimes think that one should step back and absorb before one speaks, which doesn't come easy to me.

*Given that we live in a society where our proportion of old people is increasing, do you see that as a problem?*
Well, I feel quite strongly about this: the way in which the elderly are quite often pushed aside—for instance, financially. In Australia at the moment, if you don't have anything, you get a pension. If you have saved all your life and been thrifty, you are penalised. There is no provision made, as there is in Europe, for older people's investments to be interest free. Therefore, on the one hand the government is saying, 'There's going to be more and more people you've got to look after.' But nobody is helping old people to look after themselves. There's no incentive to save money. You get provisional tax on your savings when you're generating your income from your own investments. There are all sorts of things that could be done to help old people. The cut-off point means that an awful lot of old people are really having it hard, and are pushed into homes because it's all too boring to look after them.

And that takes one right back to my feeling that the family is the most important unit in society, and to break it down is criminal. We should be building it up and looking after our old folk, because they are the people who've contributed to what we have now. Unfortunately, a lot of the elderly now are those people who grew up with no welfare, went through two world wars, and yet they are being penalised. I can't justify in my mind an elderly couple or person having a worse way of life now that they are old than when they were working.

*Is there anything about getting older that you don't like?*
Oh yes, just the physical lack of stamina. I think I'm fairly healthy and have quite a lot of energy, but I realise now that I couldn't do a five-

minute dance routine without puffing a lot, even if I managed to get to the end of it. I don't want long sleep as I did when I was young. But if I have to go out late at night and I've woken up early in the morning, I just feel much better if I can get half an hour's sleep somewhere during the day. So far I have been lucky, because I don't put on huge amounts of weight; so I haven't had to diet.

*Do you work at being fit?*
No, I don't. That's why I'm lucky. I don't exercise. I should. I feel everything will drop to the floor at any minute, but I am fairly energetic. I move around quickly, and pound up and down the stairs, and swim when I can—not for the exercise, but because I just love it. I don't sit down much.

*Has change in your physical appearance worried you? Do you look at yourself in the mirror and think, 'Oh God, I'm getting older.'?*
Yes, yes. I don't spend a lot of time, thank God, looking at myself in the mirror, but it is sometimes a shock when you see yourself unexpectedly—say you have just been talking to your daughter, and you look at yourself in the mirror, and automatically expect to look like she looks. And, of course, you don't, so you think, 'Oh God!' On the other hand, one of the loveliest things that I have seen is somebody who is growing old gracefully. I remember a dinner party in Kenya, where there was this woman who must have been in her mid-seventies when we were all in our thirties, so she did seem very old to us. But she was so full of personality and so interesting that the whole table was just riveted. You could take all the young girls in the room and leave them for dead.

*Do you tell people your age?*
I tell my friends. I don't really feel ashamed of being the age I am. What bugs me is that as an actor it's important. People put you into slots. In fact, everybody puts people into slots. You hear people come on radio saying, 'Oh, of course I'm sixty-five,' as though they should apologise for their age. I don't think one should apologise. I think one should be pleased that one has got this far, and is still hopefully functioning, and has a family and friends and a good life. I'm not ashamed of my age, only coy about my age where it's in my work scene.

*Would you ever consider having a face lift?*

Oh, yes. I'd do anything to make myself... that's not true... I wouldn't do anything. But I don't think there's anything morally wrong in making the best of what you have. My hair, I had to tint for work purposes; then when I went back dark it looked awful, so I've stayed the same colouring because it suits me. I don't think there's anything wrong with that. And if I decided that I would look better—if I could get the courage together to do it—I mean, if you feel your teeth need attention, you have them seen to. And if you feel you're too chubby, you do something to lose weight. So, yes, I would if I felt it was going to be good, yes.

*Are you frightened of death?*

No, I'm not frightened of death; only resenting it. I feel I've got so many things I want to do before my time comes. But I do sometimes fear becoming incapacitated and getting to a stage where I am not in control of my own life, either mentally or physically. I would hate that. I'm a firm believer in euthanasia. We say women should be able to have abortions because it's their bodies. Well, it's my body, and when I have finished with it, and I think I've had enough, I should be able to take that decision. After all, it's the quality of your life: it's not just living and living. If your quality goes and you're in pain, stuck in a wheel chair or in a hospital bed, and there's nothing to it any more, then I would like somebody to give me an injection or a pill and quietly go to sleep.

*Do you have any religious beliefs?*

Well, I was brought up Church of England. I'm not an ardent churchgoer, but I suppose I go to church about once every six weeks, or two months. I enjoy that. I am a Christian; yes, quite definitely. I do believe in Jesus, and I get a great deal of comfort out of that. But it's in a very unorthodox way. I think that Jesus was a really tough Israeli peasant, and I don't see him as an effete medieval-type gentleman. I think what he did was quite extraordinary. And really it was a very simple philosophy, and if we could follow just the ten commandments, the world would be a better place.

*Do you feel you have any personal relationship with God?*

Well, I feel that he really was who he said he was; otherwise he was mad, and I don't think he was mad. Or he was a charlatan, and I don't think he was a charlatan. And no one has explained to me yet if the world didn't start by some amazing creation, then how did it start? You can have all the big bangs in the world, but where did the big bangs come from? You can have it started from outer space or splitting up, but where did that come from? The simple explanation of Christianity, I find I can live with that; and then you have almost got to follow it through and believe in the life after death. But I don't envisage us all sitting up there in heaven, and you swanning through with wings on and a lovely long white dress, clutching a golden microphone. I don't really know what I feel, but I am ready to take something on faith.

*Has having children been important for you?*
Oh, yes. I look at them sometimes and think how rich we would have been if we hadn't had them, but that's a passing whim! Oh no, I love my children. I think your children enrich you and give you a feeling of continuity, that you are part of something much bigger than just yourself. I can't think of anything worse than being an isolated human being in this world. That's why I feel for all these children who don't have families, who are runaways. They're not part of anything.

You know, I can look back and think about my grandparents and my great-grandparents—who I am told came from Ireland on my father's side—and I reckon if I went over to Ireland I'd find all those roots going back. That's all important, and one's children are a part of that. Having just got our first little grandson, I often find myself wondering what his world will be like. It is like being part of a big wheel. Children are important, and they teach you a lot. I would have been a much more selfish person without my children. And your children are so honest, they make you think. Luckily, we're all good friends. If I was left with my generation I wouldn't have such a broad spectrum of life and thoughts.

*And marriage?*
[Laughs] It has definitely affected the way I think. You can't live with another human being for years and years without them influencing your thoughts. But as you get older it is very comforting to have someone whom you know so well, and who knows you so well, still there with you. And if you have the same children together, it's a very

secure feeling. That's not to say that it's easy or that it's all beds of roses; but as you get older, to have a partner that you can just be completely yourself with is comforting. Certainly, I think if marriage works, it's the best way to be.

*Clearly the way it works depends quite a lot on what people put in to it?*

I mean, we couldn't be more opposite. If we were in an arranged marriage we wouldn't even have been considered in the same breath. Robert's background, my background—totally different. Robert's upbringing and education—totally different. His world of agriculture, animals, professionalism, science—and mine of theatre and very little education in the formal sense, plus being male and female on top of all that. So certainly we have battled our way through our marriage, and we've had the most awful differences and unhappy times where we've been out of synchronisation. But we've also had lovely times. And that's something age gives. If you are here long enough, it's like being through a huge storm, and suddenly coming into a harbour where it's calm. It sounds smug to say you've made it, but there's a comfort you have, and you get the payback for the fight to get there.

Gosh, one can only talk for oneself, because marriage is so personal, but I think that to make a marriage succeed, one of the fundamental things is that you've both got to believe enormously in marriage. I've seen my mother and father very unhappy; but certainly my family had stable marriages, and my grandparents, and my husband's family the same, very stable marriages and background; and all that helps you to persevere. It's familiar. It's not familiar to have divorces, and rush off and do your own thing. And so you're apt to cling to what you know; and, in clinging, I suppose you just get stronger at it, and better at it and, if it works, that's great. I think everyone has to find their own key. With all our differences, Robert and I both felt the same: that marriage was worth fighting for and making work, and also it provided a stable background in which to bring up children, and therefore was better for them. So that with all that hoohah round the edges of not agreeing, we agreed on those fundamental things. That helps.

*When you die, how would you like to be remembered?*

What a terrible question. I'd like to be remembered with a smile, in the sense that I'd like people to remember the happy times we'd shared.

I'd like my children to remember the fun things that we've done together, and the laughs we've had. And I'd like Robert and my children to be aware—it sounds soppy, really—of how much I loved them, and what a joy they were to me.

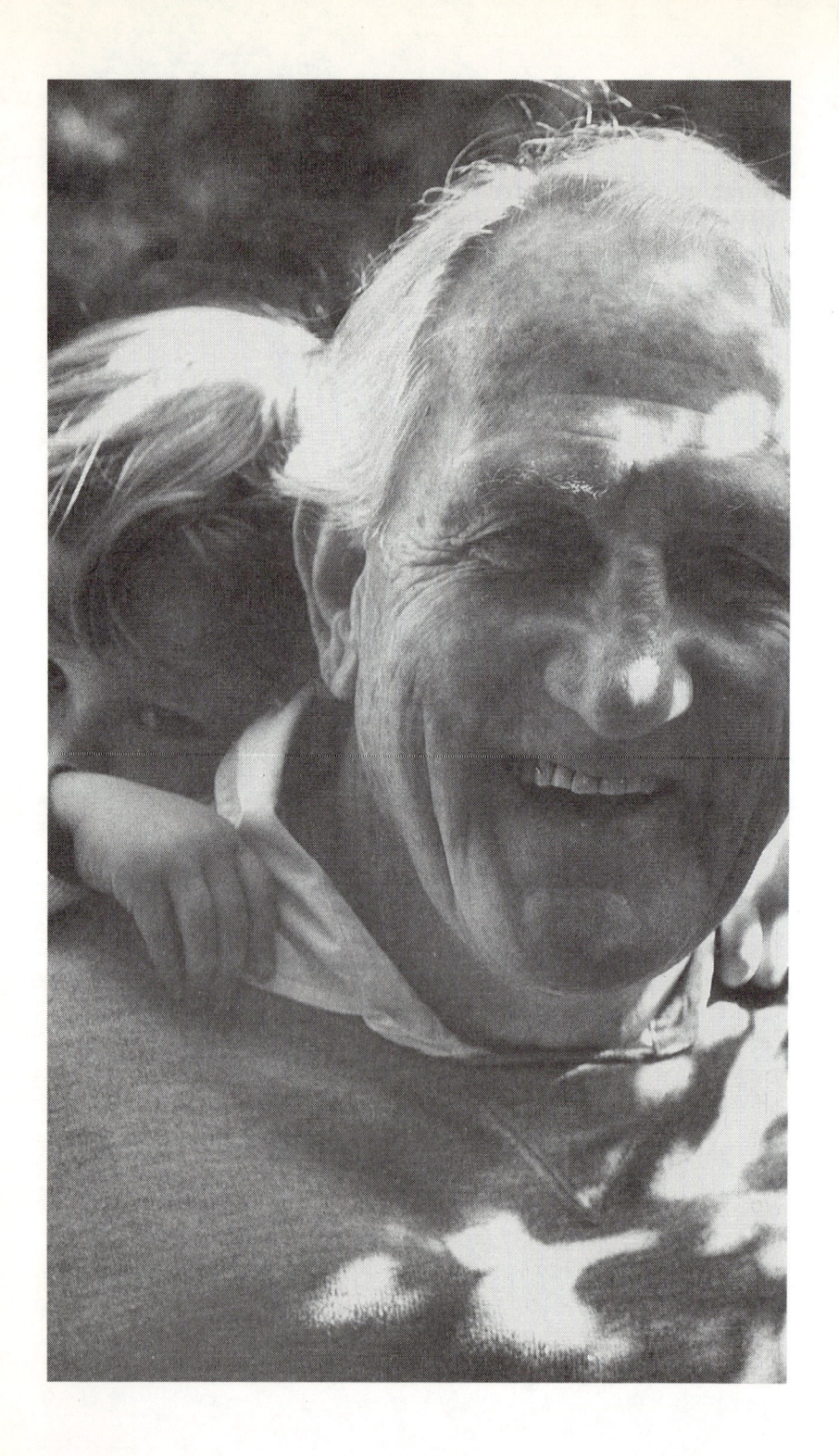

# Tom Uren
*Giving is the greatest form of loving*

Tom Uren, Labour member of parliament for over thirty years and minister in the Whitlam government, was born in Sydney's Balmain on 28 May 1921. He left school at thirteen to help his parents during the Depression years. At the age of twenty-one, he became a prisoner of the Japanese and worked on the notorious Burma-Thailand railway. Many years later, he was jailed over his campaign against Australia's involvement in Vietnam, and again for protesting against Queensland's ban on street marches.

As Minister for Urban and Regional Development in the Whitlam Government, he left a legacy of urban renewal for low-cost housing, decentralisation, the rehabilitation of Fremantle and parts of Hobart, improvements in urban public transport, and the greening of western Sydney. In 1993, Uren was made a life member of the Australian Labor Party, and an officer of the Order of Australia for service to the Australian Parliament, to urban and regional development, the environment, and the community.

Tom Uren returned to live in Balmain in circumstances which many people might have found difficult. When his new and much-loved house was first built, it ended up costing more than he could afford; so he leased the top half and lived in a make-shift dwelling underneath. The foundation pillars were hung with Lloyd Rees paintings and the works of other fine Australian artists; his washing was strung in between; and opera would soar forth from speakers hitched to the floor joists.

'It's such a lovely house, I just enjoy it all,' he said. This is not unlike his attitude to ageing—'It's such a lovely life, I enjoy it all.' He now occupies the entire house, with his wife Christine Logan, who is a singer with the Australian Opera, and her three-year-old daughter, Ruby.

My wife died in 1981. I had a long relationship with a younger person that I married recently; but it was an on-and-off thing for a number of years, and that always has a hurt when older men are in love with younger women. It sometimes upsets you, but I must say the last three years has been really just bliss. It's just wonderful. She tends to love me as much if not more than I love her. Love's generally never an equal thing; but, be that as it may, I'm extremely happy. Christine is a real giver, and she's got a great deal of the qualities my wife Patricia had.

My wife, Patricia, was probably the nicest human being I ever met or have ever known. She had a great inner beauty about her. And Christine Logan has a similar inner beauty. She is loved by people, and she has a real warmth. I think it is because I love her baby Ruby so much that she tends to love me. Ruby is three years old now. We split up for a little while, but we got back together again while Christine was still pregnant; so I was with her most of time that she carried that pregnancy. I'm proud of that. My first two children were adopted, so I understand how adopted children need extra love. I'm not in competition with the real father; he's got a good relationship with Christine, and sees the child every week, and that's working out fine. I'm happy about that.

*Tom, you're quite a bit older than Christine, aren't you?*

Yes, thirty years plus.

*So did that give you cause for concern?*

No, it never did. Christine always said she'd never found an age difference between us—except I always knew what I wanted; she didn't know what she wanted. I wanted to take the responsibilities of looking after her and Ruby because I love them both. But she made the decision about marriage, and I'm pleased.

*Are you still as committed today?*

Yes, yes. I think I'm probably as committed today as I've ever been in my whole life. Sometimes it makes me very sad to see society so individualistic, particularly market forces. I think that's the law of the jungle, and I've fought that all my life. I've always been a collectivist, but with age you get a kind of patience and you see a broader picture. You can look at yourself as well as looking at others, and I don't get as adamant in my criticisms. For instance, getting the life membership of the Labor Party, there were about thirty-odd people who got it the same time as I did, and the applause was always polite; but when it came to me it was nearly a standing ovation of the whole conference. New South Wales right machine: they've never had any love or joy for me in the past. I've gone to the mike when prominent right-wing people have hissed me—their venom for me was so strong—but that's mellowed, and there seems to be a broader acceptance.

Even the establishment seem to accept me for what I am, perhaps because I have been consistent. I fought Packer for six-and-a-half years in every court in the land. I fought both Packer and Fairfax together, but the longest one was against Packer. I just wouldn't give in. I used the money that I got from Fairfax to finance me in my fight with Packer. You're made a certain way; you don't have to boast about it. I've never been frightened about physical courage in war or peace, but I think I've always had more moral courage than physical courage.

*Is there anything that does frighten you?*
The only thing that ever did frighten me was cholera when I was on the Burma-Thailand railway. But in the middle Sixties I walked across a 'line of freedom', and from that point on I've never allowed anybody or any system to intimidate me. Once I walked across that line, I continued to grow. I didn't carry any guilt if I had extra sexual relationships. I would never do it to hurt; but when you are away from your wife for a long time, particularly in political life, sometimes it happens. And I would carry a lot of guilt. I think I became more sexually free, but I also became politically and morally free. I'm one of the few that stood up to Whitlam in the Whitlam years. He was a very dominating prime minister, a commanding prime minister; but I always stood my ground, just as I stood my ground against Hawke. I did the same when I was a Woolworths manager: I stood up against the system. I enjoyed my life very much as a Woolworths manager; it was a wonderful part of my life.

*When you've taken those stands, have you ever been wrong?*
[Laughter] Oh probably, but I made the stand for better for worse. I'm sure I was wrong in making the strong decision for Cairns becoming treasurer. It was a strong moral position on my part. Jimmy was never really keen to take on treasury, but both Gwen Cairns and I wanted

him to take it, so he did. I think that I expected too much of him, and I pushed him too much. His relationship with Morosi was his downfall, but he was in love. He's never really admitted that, but in the end he put Morosi before our party, and he put her before even the Left of the party—even though you have to recognise that up until at least the Christmas of l974, moving into 1975, he was revered by the nation. He went to Darwin for Cyclone Tracey, and the nation loved him for his great compassion. He's a very beautiful human being, Cairns. I can't say that I've loved too many other politicians in my lifetime, but I've a great love for Cairns.

*In this case it seemed as if he made a decision about his personal life that had a huge impact on his career and on his party. How do you weigh that kind of decision? Have you always put your party politics ahead of your personal relationships?*

Like I've already admitted, I'm not a promiscuous person and I never was a promiscuous man. But I did it in a discreet way, and I would do that because I wouldn't want my class enemies to use that against my own party. I always felt that I was a representative of my class. I never put tickets on myself, but I served the national Left and I served the nation as a whole. I've never seen myself ever in the pre-eminent position of, say, a Cairns or a Whitlam. I've always found myself as just Tom Uren doing my work. For the first eleven years I was in parliament, I didn't even run for any executive position. When I did stand, and was elected, to my great surprise Whitlam gave me something which was nearest to his heart—and that was Urban and Regional Development. That was my other great commitment. I was the first national spokesperson the Labor Party ever had on the environment. That just grew out of me: my love for my environment and an extension of my love for the human race.

I suppose they were many of the things that Weary Dunlop had given me, travelling and working with him in prison camps. I was just one of his boys, one of his thousand on that Hintock mountain camp. Weary arrived about a week before we did on the Burma-Thailand railway. I walked into his camp on the 26 January 1943, and remained with him until after the railway line had been completed. I served under him the whole of those eighteen months, and we remained very close. When I was elected to parliament, he was proud because I was one of his boys. Even recently, a few days before he died, he wrote and told me how proud he was of me and my role in history, and so forth. He's been a wonderful part in my life. But I've had a lot of wonderful people in my life: Roosevelt encouraged me into politics with his New Deal policy ... the great influence of my mother when I was growing up.

*Tell me about this part of your life.*
I was born and lived in Balmain, which in those early days had a big social impact. Of course, we rented a house, and I can remember it just as if it was yesterday. My mother would talk to me when I was a young boy, telling me about having to pay rent. When the landlord came, he would ask if there was anything else my mother could pawn to pay the rent. A lot of people aren't aware of this: but in the 1920s, if people were out of work, they had to go before the 'nice' people of the community, the so-called elite, to see if they were worthy of welfare. Those things remained in my heart the whole of my lifetime. My mother would get embarrassed when I'd mention these things in later years, but she didn't realise how she'd sown that seed of social feeling in my early years.

*Were you a large family?*
Three boys. I had an older brother, Jack, and a younger brother, Les; so it wasn't a big family. My father was in and out of work, with long periods when he couldn't get a job. He was quite a skilled person but without any qualifications, so he'd always have to do the hard, laborious work. When he could, he would work as a labourer in boat building, but he would also build boats himself. He was a very small man—he'd been a jockey—but not short; about five foot eight.

*Was this a happy childhood?*
Yes, because my mother was a very loving woman. I suppose, really, I'm a product of my mother more than my father, although I was very proud of my father, particularly the way he died. He had a tumour on the brain, and I've never seen a person die with so much courage. I'd seen so many people die in prison camp, and it was the way in which they died: some people die like curs; others die like heroes. My father was a hero.

*Were you clever at school?*
No. I don't think I was bright; I was tenacious. I always asked questions

and I was always interested in history, geography, and maths, but found it very difficult to deal with English and grammar. I seem to write a lot of letters to the *Sydney Morning Herald* just the same, but I've had to struggle with my diction and grammar all my life.

*Were you a boxer?*
Yes. In my army days I started doing that.

*Given your love of peace, how do you equate the two?*
Well, it was a bit of an embarrassment all my life. But I was always more involved with the skill of boxing than the brutality of boxing, and believed that if a man has got the ability to box, it's his responsibility to look after the fellow who can't. It disappoints me when I see thugs in the ring. If you're a gentleman in the ring, you're a gentleman outside the ring. I always was more interested in that type of boxing.

*Tom, when you were on the Burma Railway, did you at any stage think you mightn't make it?*
The only time that I didn't think I would make it was during the cholera epidemics. Otherwise, I always thought I'd make it. I always had great faith, until in the middle sixties I made the decision that I wasn't a Christian any more; but because I found those beautiful stories of Christ moved me tremendously, I questioned what had made me emotionally involved. The only thing I could put it down to was my commitment to other human beings. I've always treated Jesus Christ as a man of good will. You've got to have love and commitment to the human race, and seek to make a better world. I like to quote Martin Luther King when he said, 'Hate distorts the personality and scars the soul. It is more injurious to the hater than the hated.'

*Then idealism is still strong within you?*
Yes. It's even stronger today. But you've got to recognise that, within the West as well as the East, bureaucrats are people who have really tried to frustrate and clog up the system. Sometimes you have to take them on. For instance, the anti-march laws against Bjelke-Petersen: our weapon was to put that many people in jail by putting them before the magistrates, refusing to pay their bail or fines, and clogging up the system, so that the police and court system would recognise that immoral and unjust laws cannot be maintained.

*But how is that we keep throwing up systems that become totalitarian?*

I wouldn't use the word 'totalitarian' so much in the West; but 'authoritarian,' 'bureaucratic,' and 'elitist'. And for that you've got to fight the system. Freedom isn't something you can say, 'Look, I've got it!' You've got to continually protect it for ever more. In my last speech I made in parliament, I said that my commitment would be to the anti-war movement, to the human rights movement, and to the environmental movement. A lot of people say to me, 'Where are the revolutionaries of today?' The young people in Greenpeace, the conservation groups, and in Amnesty International: these are the great crusaders, the people who are standing up for real freedoms, and we should be proud of them. I'm a born optimist, and I think that good can overcome evil.

*Do you have any kind of philosophy about where good comes from?*

Even though I've moved away from Christianity, the great philosophers like Martin Luther King and Pope John XXIII have influenced me with their values very much. And Friere—even though he's a Marxist, he's also a Catholic. So I've got a lot of Christian values that I cherish. We have to stand up for people and issues when we see good, even if they come from conservative people. For instance, I'm extremely proud of Malcolm Fraser: first of all in his stand in Africa, and secondly his stand as head of Care Australia. He's doing a tremendous job. I have that warmth and affection for Whitlam, and I have the same thing with Fraser. I'm critical of Gough's position on East Timor, but apart from that we have practically full agreement on most issues nowadays. I find he's a real comrade-in-arms.

*Do you think there is any life after death?*

Well, I did move to an atheist position, but I wouldn't like to preach my view about that. For instance, I'm so happy I was walking past Dorothy McMahon's Congregational church in Pitt Street, Sydney.

*You are moved; why are there tears in your eyes?*

It's the feeling that she's a good person. Her church door was open, and I just went in to meditate and said to myself, 'Well, somebody has been good to me'. It gives me strength. I really do believe that we have evolved; and a part of that progressing is to feel secure not only within yourself but within your nation, and that nation has to look towards other nations. Even though I'm a proud Australian national, I talk about the universe, and I talk about the human race. You know what Martin Luther King said, that 'injustice anywhere is a threat to justice everywhere'. You can't ignore it.

I believe that Keating's statement of 2 December 1992, at Redfern Park, will eventually be one of the great documents of an Australian political leader—to have the guts and determination to make an admission of guilt of what we have done to those unfortunate people, the aboriginal people who we have exploited for so long. Weary Dunlop, this wonderful man with such a conservative background, collectivised our wealth in a prison camp, and worked on a simple philosophy of the strong looking after the weak, the young looking after the old, and the fit looking after the sick. He would send our blokes out to barter with the Chinese and Thai traders, and they would bring back drugs and food to look after the sick and the needy. I still believe that in a society like ours we should be much more collective.

I was critical of the Hawke government, and I was critical of Paul Keating as a treasurer. But I was supportive of Paul Keating becoming prime minister. I could see that there was something special in the attitude of this man, who's got such wonderful and remarkable eyes that are the window of his soul; there is something inherently decent in Keating. Given the opportunity to lead his nation, he could prove to become one of our great prime ministers. He could be more collective, and less elitist, but I think there is something great and wonderful about him. He's got a lot of Whitlam in him. I feel Keating will continue to grow in understanding of the ordinary people's problems.

You've got no idea of how critical I was of the Hawke government for refusing to do anything for the social and physical infrastructures of our cities. I warned our people behind the scenes. I said, 'There's going to be an explosion in the western suburbs of Sydney, and when it comes it's going to be the fault of governments. It's passive at present, but have no doubt it could turn very ugly in the future unless we do something about it.' Whitlam had a bigness about him. Whitlam created things.

*Are you saying there was a lack of vision within the Hawke government?*

Yes. It was free market forces in government [rising voice]: 'You can't have a vision for the future! It costs money!'

*Tom, is it hard for you not to think of politics all the time?*
Well, I love my music, and I love theatre and opera. I am a late learner in all these things. I love the environment, but I am very greatly influenced by Barry Commoner. The first principle of the environment is that everything is connected to everything else; and the second principle is that everything has got to go somewhere. I find this interrelationship so much in living. For instance, if I go to a party or a group of friends, I don't try to impose my views, because everybody tends to know what my views are. But if I find anybody putting a royalist line, I'm in there; I give him a straight left and a right under the ribs in a friendly sort of way.

*Does it worry you at all getting older?*
No, no. First of all, I'll go when I've got to go. I am concerned that I'm never a burden on any of my loved ones; that's why for a long time I've been conscious of my health and what I eat. I was a fairly big meat-eater in my younger days, but now I rarely eat meat. I'm guided by Pritikin, but I'm not dogmatic about it. I eat mostly pastas and brown rice, fresh fruit, and things of that description; a little bit of white meat and a little bit of fish, a lot of coarse bread.

I'm in good health. The only thing is that I've got a pretty rickety old spine which my POW days left me, and I can't do any physical work much. I continually do exercises to strengthen the muscles in my back. I don't own a car. I walk a lot, I use public transport, and that gives me communication with people as well. On the ferries, the buses, the trains, or on the streets, the great thing in my life is the rewards I get from people, just that greeting of their eyes. I find that giving is the greatest reward of living. You know, with all Packer's millions, you can't buy those smiles, those greetings of peoples' eyes saying, 'How are you, Tom?' It's that warmth that people give you that's the great joy of living.

*What happens when people let you down?*
Well, if I've got a good strong relationship with a person, and I think they've done the wrong thing, I phone them up. I don't try to cover it over. I just say, 'Well, I disagree with what you've done.' For instance, I told some of my parliamentary colleagues in no uncertain terms what I thought of them in the Gulf war. It was the principle of sending our young men to war, thinking that war can be the solution to international

conflict. I was proud that ten people of that caucus, and a big percentage of them women, stood up and said, 'I won't vote for our government's decision to send our young men to war,' and walked out of the parliament.

*Are there advantages in getting older?*
There is the point, particularly when you're overseas and they say, 'Are you over sixty or sixty-five?' I've been to most of the great galleries of the world, and I am admitted for half-price.

*Are there disadvantages?*
No, I don't find any disadvantages. Even at my age, seventy-two years young, I feel very sad that we've got so many single mothers struggling to exist, we've so many people unemployed in our community, and my heart goes out to them. I've never been a charity worker, and I don't want to start at my age. I've been a person that fought for equity and justice.

*Are there things you still want to do?*
Yes, I'd like to see a more progressive, just, democratic, and a freer government coming through in our society. I'm the type of person who struggles for the loaf of bread; and if I can't get the loaf of bread, in the end I'm grateful for the crumbs that fall from the table. But it's a continuous struggle. I think the women's movement is one of the great hopes of our whole world scene. When I took my anti-war position on the Iraq war, I travelled round Australia, and in every meeting—without exception—a woman was the organiser of the anti-war movement. It was quite remarkable. Women have always been more compassionate about war and peace. There are, of course, some women—they are easily identifiable—that try to outdo the men. But generally women have got their own special persuasion about them.

*Has it ever been difficult for you on a personal level—because much about what the women's movement stands for challenges men?*
No. I'd say that with most women in the labour movement, those on the Left, I've always been fairly close to them. Probably it's been the influence of my mother. Mum wanted a daughter, and I'd say, 'Oh mum, I'm the woman in the family.' Like all of us, I'm a male chauvinist, and I've got to examine and re-examine myself every day; as I've got

to do it on racism, also. If you really are fair dinkum about combating the questions of sexism, you've first of all got to look at yourself in every facet of your life. You've got to look at your relationships both with your own wife and with other women. I do the same thing with racism. You've got to examine and re-examine yourself if you are to progress and grow. You've got to feel in your heart that you are right, and then have the guts to go out and fight for it. Uren has to be happy with Uren. It is the way I am.

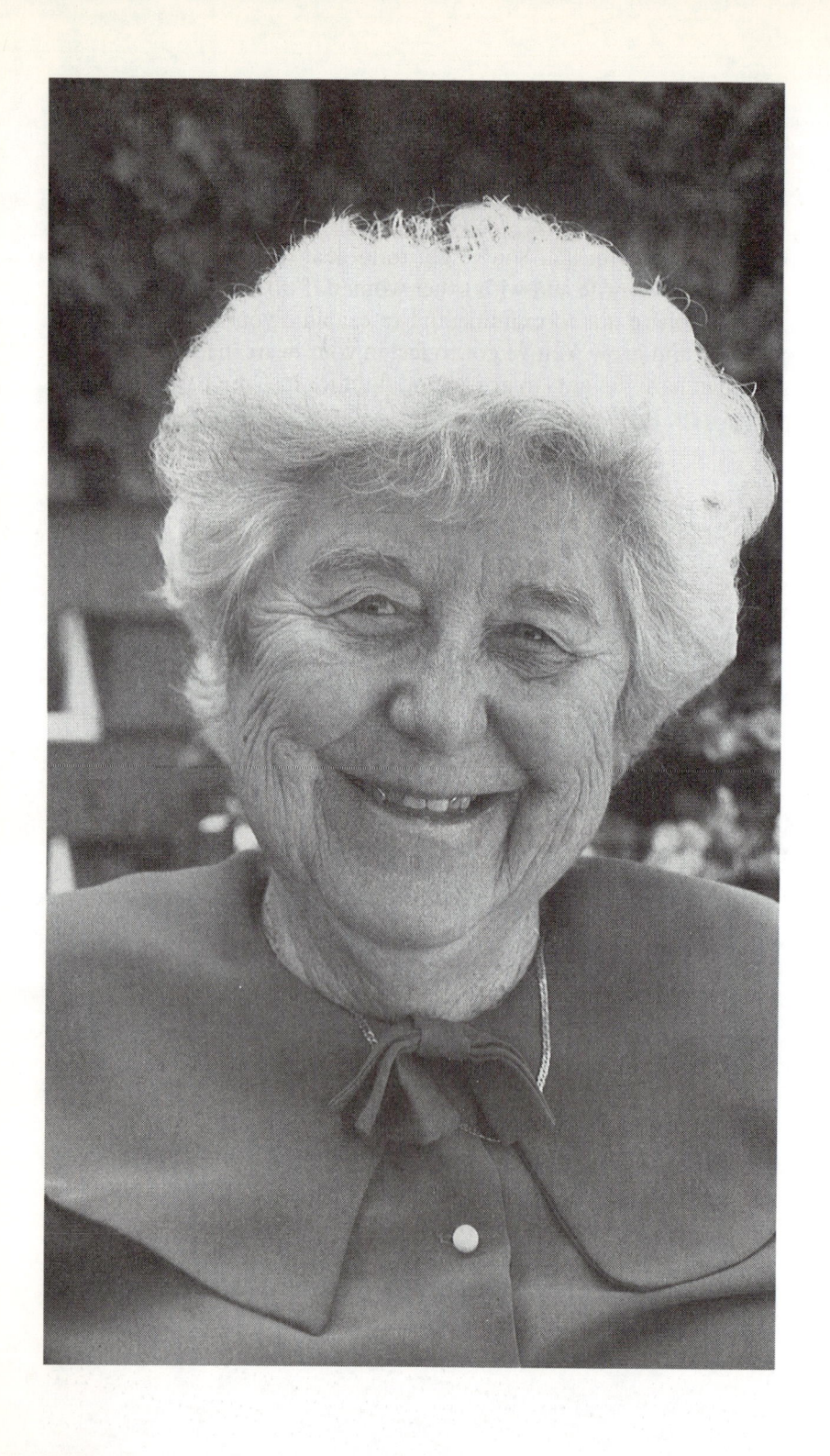

# Noreen Hewett
*My life has been magnificent*

Noreen Hewett is a tireless worker on behalf of older women. She helped found the Older Women's Network in New South Wales, and now works there nearly all the time. The Network is a grassroots organisation with a commitment to the belief that older women are the real experts in matters concerning their lives. It provides a range of services and activities, including a lively theatre group. Members are skilled lobbyists on policy issues affecting older women; similar networks have been set up around Australia.

Hewett says the reason for a network specifically for older women is that women age differently from men. They have different health needs, are more likely than men to be living in poverty and alone in old age, and their special needs are often ignored. Ask Hewett why not a network for men, and she replies, 'If men wish to set up a network for themselves, they are welcome to do it.'

Noreen Hewett was born in Sydney in May 1920, and has served on numbers of organisations affecting people's lives—ranging from working in progress associations to being national secretary of the Australian Pensioners' Federation. She has also been a member of the Social Security Advisory council, and a member of the NSW Medical Board.

I live in a block of units. I've got a little tiny unit and, oh, lots of things happen in units. Units can be little boxes of separated people living terribly lonely lives; on the other hand, they can also be communities. In my particular block, there was a Hungarian woman who lived alone, and she ended up becoming so confused she had to be admitted to a psychiatric hospital. Her problem was malnutrition, because she couldn't be bothered to eat. It wasn't that she had no money. She was lonely. Although she was physically mobile, she was given meals on wheels for a while as a way of changing her patterns. And people would say, 'Why should she be getting meals on wheels? However, meals on wheels and a little more communication with neighbours changed her eating habits, and now she's a woman with much more vitality, even though she's very aged.

A similar thing happened to a friend of mine. At first they thought she had Alzheimer's, but subsequently they diagnosed her as having malnutrition. A woman who had enough money to live comfortably had malnutrition because she was a woman who couldn't be bothered cooking for herself, despite all her knowledge of the culinary arts.

*Why do you think this extreme loneliness happens? Is it mainly women whose partners die and suddenly they are coping on their own?*

Sometimes. That Hungarian woman, her husband had died some time ago. She seemed to be all right, and then she acquired a new partner, which I thought was wonderful. She had him living with her for some time and then he died, too, quite suddenly; and it was after that she became ill. My friend, who was such a good cook, finally struck up an acquaintance with an unemployed fellow who lived in the same units, and she ended up cooking for him. He had a car, so he took her out. It was a good exchange.

The other thing that often happens to women is that there are social pressures from neighbours about how they should behave. There was another woman in my unit (it's like 'Number 96'!) who was a librarian, and her husband had a stroke. They were both Hungarian, and she was looked down upon by the neighbours because at first she didn't leave work. Work was tremendously important to her. I said to her she shouldn't feel that she had to be home; they had a bit of money, why didn't she buy in the services that were needed? But in the event she left work. She was desperately unhappy, desperately depressed, and she ended up having a heart attack and dying before her husband, simply because of prejudice and a lack of support.

*Can we talk about the stereotypes attached to older women?*
Yes. The fact that men retire but women don't. They're expected to carry on all those nurturing roles for the rest of their lives. Women are still grandmas or mums, whereas a man achieves some self-worth or identity through his work. Very often, the woman's work was seen just as a diversion from her other responsibilities. In spite of all the modern attempts at liberating women, it's only now that older women are making their push for an equality and a right of identity. Another fact is that the majority of volunteering is done by women, and by older women when it comes to older people's services. That's definitely stereotyping. What else?

*Appearance is a big one, isn't it? The fact that we have a culture where you're not allowed to get old if you're a woman, and that can be very demoralising.*
The need to be attractive to the man has enormous impact, even on people who according to stereotype notions were quite beautiful but still felt ugly or inadequate in terms of their physical appearance. I think a lot of older women now feel, 'Well I've done with all that; I don't have to be in this sort of environment of trying any more.' And so I feel more comfortable with my older body than I did when I was younger.

*Was this a gradual transition, or did you try to fight getting older?*
I don't think I ever fought getting older. But like a lot of other people—even within our own organisation—to be called old was seen as an insult. Whereas now I feel I can wear that tag with pride. Many people still shy away from it, and there's a lot of discussion now about the International Day of the Elderly. You mustn't call it the International Day of the Elderly. In some respects 'elderly' is seen as old, old, old. But whether it's a label or not, I see it as a fact of life that one accepts chronological age and some biological differences in age, and then looks at the benefits. Because there are benefits.

*Tell me about some of the benefits.*
I think women have a lot of pressures when they're younger. To be post menopausal has a lot of compensation, even sexually. I had in

many ways a better sexual life after menopause when I felt freer from all those things that used to happen to my body, including the fear of becoming pregnant. Even though one might have wrinkles and some arthritic condition, a lot of women still feel more comfortable and still feel relatively well. A lot of the time when I was younger I was working under stress in a job, and coping with a family. I'm not doing this any longer. I'm better in many ways—physically, mentally—freer from the boss, from having to do all the things that you might object to personally because you're working for a wage and helping somebody else to be efficient. To be able to do your own thing is wonderful. There still are demands put upon you, from the family and what-have-you, but there's a voluntariness about it that's not there when you're younger.

***Freedom to be yourself in the sense of not conforming, if that's the way you wish to be?***

I think I've become more outrageous. I've got a sister-in-law who's always apprehensive of what I'm going to say in company, particularly to younger people—that I might talk about sexuality or things that might seem quite inappropriate for a person of my age. But I don't find any inappropriateness whatsoever. I find that I have quite a rapport with younger people, and that I meet them on equal terms—not even from the position of the wise old elder (although I think there is a lot of wisdom in old age) but merely as a person. One of the good things about younger people is that they can accept this. There's often not the same barrier of, 'You shouldn't be talking like that.' Even in dress. I'm dressed up today, but that's because I'm going somewhere formal later; but normally I'm casual. Again, my sister-in-law—she and I are great mates, but we're so different. She thinks that she must get dressed up to go down the street still, and I go down in tracksuit and joggers.

***Are you married still, or are you widowed?***

I'm widowed, and that was a different life. In one of the workshops that we held earlier, we had one on housing, and we asked people to say their greatest fears. My greatest fear was living alone. Never in my whole life had I lived alone. Never, always with a lot of extended family, and so on. So that was a terrible prospect for me; but I must say one gets used to it providing you have these other interests like I have. In fact, I sometimes think I'd like more time alone just to do all the things I don't do in company. Even to be able to read and look at silly programmes on TV. But I do think that people need an interest—it doesn't matter what it is—and women flourish when they find it.

*One of the stereotypes in our society is that you cease to have sexual desires, beginning post-menopause, and absolutely by the time you're sixty, seventy, or eighty.*

I certainly had a lot more sexual satisfaction in my later life, and it continued right up until about two years before my husband died. Part of sexuality is touching, comforting, and holding, and so we had that. When I listen to other women, I think that I had a fairly satisfactory sexual relationship; and after he died, I still felt sexual feelings. There even were approaches from a couple of men, but I didn't want that sort of tie. And I just found ways myself not to actually satisfy but to accommodate my sexual desires. So that still happens. I try to stimulate conversation about sex between peers, but a lot of women are not ready to acknowledge that they are still sexual beings when in fact they are. Some friends considered that I am a very highly sexed person, because I loved my husband's body. I loved it. I'm sure he enjoyed mine. His gift to me was the confidence of feeling loved. So that sort of frankness I think is healthy, and I think it's unhealthy not to admit your sexuality at an older age or even to enjoy it.

*Have you seen people in love when they're in their seventies, eighties?*

Yes, I've seen people of much older ages fall in love and acquire sexual partners. I think that's good and healthy and increasing. We're all a product of change in our society; and older people change, too. And so there are more people who don't conform to past patterns of getting married and then finding a completely unsatisfactory partnership. Now they experiment and find greater freedom within partnerships.

*How do you think we rate as a society in our attitudes to old age?*

I think our society has lots and lots and lots to learn about old age. There's fear of old age happening to oneself, and there's objectifying of it. Even studies that are undertaken of people in older age don't involve the people themselves, don't really respect their opinions and input into shaping the sort of society that we ought to be developing. Generally, older people are excluded as though they've had it. They're here, but they're seen as appendages. They're waiting in God's waiting room, waiting to die. It's felt that there's only the extraordinary individual who's likely to have anything to say or any impact. So I think, by and large, there are extremely negative attitudes to old age, and I think those negative attitudes create self-images among older people that make them feel inadequate and useless.

*How is your energy?*

Great. On workshops and things like that I get on a real high. I love a contest of ideas. Don't mind a fight, actually, within organisations like the Combined Pensioners annual conferences. When I say a fight, I mean a very strong interchange on issues and policies. Intellectually bouncing off each other as we do in the workshops and developing new ideas—even strange ideas—is wonderful. Very mentally stimulating. Some of my forgetfulness may be something to do with different usage of different parts of the brain. Who knows? I'm not concerned about that; I don't feel that my intellectual capacity is diminished. Rather, that in the voluntary life I've led since retirement it has been heightened because of the huge amount of documentation that I have to read, and having to focus perhaps on something I hadn't thought of before.

*When you were younger and married, were you working outside the home?*

A lot of the time. Some of the time I was working in voluntary organisations. My husband and I never accumulated any money. He was a boiler-maker's helper in industry. I was secretarial, fairly skilled, and so sometimes I earned more money than he did. Other times, I'd leave work and do some voluntary activity.

*Children?*

Yeah. Two boys. One's actually a step-son. My husband was widowed early, and he had a boy. Intellectually, I've always been fairly non-conformist, but conditioned by work practice to a subsidiary role. I think it was a sort of intellectual drifting in regard to occupation. I envy those people who've been able to choose a career and develop within it.

*Do you think that if you had you been born into a later generation that you would have done something quite different?*

Yes I do. I left school at fourteen, after repeating third year, and I think I had four Bs. That was the exam result, so that I had a very poor formal education. Because my sister was very ill I grew up sometimes at Tempe with my grandparents, and sometimes with my parents at Guildford or Merrylands. I seemed to be good at English and writing, but not much else.

*Tell me about your childhood. What was it like?*
Well, it was funny. I lived with my grandmother a lot of the time, not only because my younger sister was very ill, but my father was a First World War veteran and he was sometimes in psychiatric institutions. He ... you know ... what did they call it, neurasthenia? He had a pension for it. But I was actually very afraid of him. I was afraid of the ... the ... his ... talking in the middle of the night, and the fact that my mother had to ... seemed to have to do everything for everybody and look after him as well. My grandmother, I adored. She was Scottish and fey and a romantic. She used to tell lots of stories, so that was the happy part of my childhood. But I wasn't terribly happy at home, because my father tried to commit suicide when I was probably about seven or eight. I was in the yard, when he was in the washhouse. I didn't even realise at the time what had happened, but years after I remembered those things and asked an aunt. Later, he was in psychiatric institutions.

*So what did he do in the washhouse?*
Cut his throat. And that gave me the idea that there was some mental problem with the family. Like most young people, I felt vulnerable and sensitive and emotional, and I always thought that probably I had an hereditary psychological problem, and so I didn't ever want to take on too much responsibility.

*Looking back on your life, do you have a sense of shape that makes sense?*
I guess so. Even though I worked in the Repat as a stenographer, and in other places, too, I was introduced to books when I was quite young—books that challenged—so I think that had a lot to do with shaping my early life. When I was about sixteen or seventeen—in 1936—the Spanish war was on, and the local librarian was putting me on to all sorts of books. Later, I became involved on the fringe of a pseudo-Bohemian set, Pakies in Elizabeth Street, frequented by writers, artists, and just some rouseabouts like me who liked to go and dance and listen to discussions. I was also introduced to theatre, and all of it was questioning, wanting something different from my own uneducated background.

*Were you politically active?*

Yes, I was. That was again through the Spanish War, and through my brother reading and bringing home books. I became a Leftist, and joined the Communist Party in the war years when it was illegal. I really didn't know anything about its politics, but I thought it would be rather exciting to belong to an illegal organisation. I did believe in socialism. I don't think I was very good at the theoretical parts of it, but later I was disgusted by the various things that were happening. I had a lot of friends, people who were very idealistic, who were also very confounded by what happened, particularly at the time of Czechoslovakia.

*What do you think has impelled you to become so active now in the Older Women's Network?*

I had a strong conviction that women, and particularly older women, had different agendas to men. That wasn't a question of hostility, it was a question of recognition. I wanted to pursue that further because I felt more comfortable working in women's organisations than in mixed organisations, although I enjoyed it all.

*You said that you were afraid of living on your own. What about now? Is there anything that you are afraid of?*

In a way, the same thing. Pleasant as it is to be able to do exactly as one likes, I feel at this stage of life that it would be good to share. Part of it is because I feel this sense of support and commonality with so many older women. And the other is that I really think it's increasingly difficult for me and other older women that I know, to live within our income. I just live on the pension with very little else. So I think that both environmentally, and just from pure economics, we would be better trying to match up; having a sense of independence but also a sharing. A lot of that's going to be experimental, but I've been talking to women who are achieving it. A lot of older people, me included, wouldn't like to have a heart attack and be left lying around for a week or so.

*Do you get frightened in the middle of the night?*

I don't now, but that's because I've built-in security to my living accommodation—bars on some windows because I live on the ground floor. But the fact is I am frightened, otherwise I'd go out at night and come home late on my own, and I don't do those things. I go out—usually with somebody—and we share a taxi home if we're going to the theatre. So I still have that fear of physical violence, particularly being mugged or being raided. Yeah, I have all those fears.

*How does that affect you? Does it make you angry?*
It makes me resentful rather than angry. I remember coming home when I was eighteen or nineteen at two o'clock in the morning, after going to a dance in town, and it didn't occur to me to be really worried. But now, if it's dark at half past eight and I'm coming home at night time, I'm really alert and apprehensive.

*Are you frightened of death?*
I don't think I am, perhaps because of having seen my husband die at very close quarters. I'd like to have control over my death. I keep procrastinating about things I ought to do, like giving someone an enduring power of attorney, and writing down all the things I want to happen—like, I don't particularly want a funeral. I want to be able to end my life and not in the ways that my father or my brother did, but rationally, sanely, so that I have control. Or, if I haven't control, that I'm helped to die. I think it's true that one has a greater acceptance of death as one grows older. I find that some very religious people are more frightened of dying, despite the fact that they're supposed to be guaranteed a happier life in the hereafter.

*So you don't have that feeling about the hereafter?*
I don't have that kind of feeling, no.

*Why don't you want a funeral?*
I just don't like the trappings of a funeral. I always say to my family, if you like to have a group of people round for drinks and say, 'Well she wasn't a bad old duck,' that's okay, but have a celebration rather than a mournful ceremony.

*What would you like to celebrate in your life?*
I'm not quite sure. I don't expect to be remembered. I feel satisfied with my life that I haven't done extremely mundane things; that I have explored beyond stereotyping, beyond conformity, even in ways that might have proved disastrous. But nevertheless I dwell at times on the magnificence of ordinary people. I know myself as an ordinary person, and I feel my life has been magnificent.

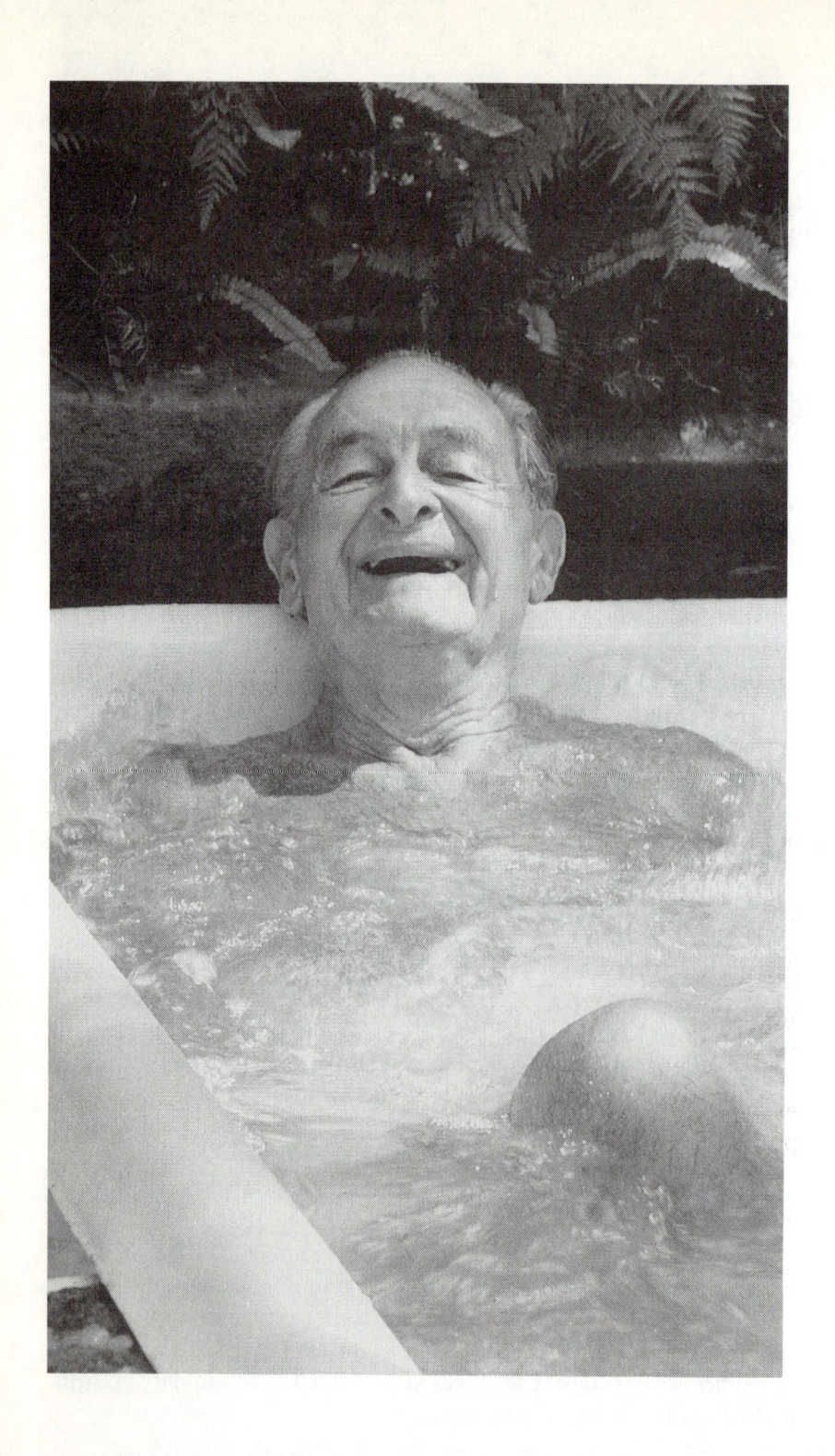

# Dick Paget-Cooke
*Bloody marvellous!*

Richard Anthony Paget-Cooke, MBE, MA, Liveryman of the Worshipful Company of Grocers, City of London, was born in England in August 1919, educated at Eton College then Christ Church, Oxford, served as a major in the Grenadier Guards, saw active service in North Africa and Italy in World War Two, and was decorated. After the war, he became a public relations consultant in England, moved to Australia in 1968, and established another successful PR career here, and was a Fellow of the Public Relations Institute of Australia. His first marriage was in England in 1944, during which he had two daughters. His second marriage was in Australia in 1975.

He has suffered for many years with arthritis, has had two hip replacements, and a recent serious illness. But, apart from the odd grimace, he dismisses his own discomforts. He lives in Pittwater with his wife, Mary, is an occasional reader on *Radio for the Print Handicapped*, maintains a lively interest in everything and everyone, and his house is frequently full of people of all ages—particularly young people.

I don't remember my childhood in a big way. I can remember looking up through the surface of the Round Pond in Kensington Gardens, having in some way fallen into it, and seeing a man poking at me with his umbrella and being hoicked out. Now, whether I really remember this, or whether it's family myth, I don't know. I was about three or four.

*Did you have a very privileged childhood?*

Yes, an aspiring one, because my parents were not blue-bloods, but my mother wanted me to go to Eton. My father said, 'No, he should go to Cheltenham, where I went.' And so the compromise was, 'If he can get a scholarship to Eton, then he can go.' I did get a scholarship, and I went.

*When you first came to Australia, was it difficult to settle?*

I came under very strange personal circumstances, involving a disastrous domestic crisis. I came on my own, and I'd left what I'd been behind. But I also came to start a public relations business. So the starting of the business was all-engrossing. I didn't know what I was doing at first, but I had to find out very quickly and I had to make it go. Also, initially there was the awful domestic crisis. I don't really want to talk about that, except to say thank goodness for two things: one, that within four to five months, the whole thing had crashed to the ground completely; and secondly—and much more importantly—I would never otherwise have met my present wife, and never have been married for over twenty years. So it was a two-edged thing.

*Has it been a good life?*

Oh, one of unbelievable good fortune and good luck. I am constantly amazed. Why I should have been allowed to have it I can't think, because I'm not an especially good sort of chap. I hope I'm not particularly bad; and yet so far, in over seventy years, it's been nearly all really good.

*Dick, are you surprised to be the age you are?*

Amazed, absolutely astonished. My father died when he was sixty-four, so I've had ten years more than him. My mother admittedly didn't die till she was eighty-seven. I don't think I necessarily identify more with my father, but I was aware that he died too early. And I'm delighted I haven't, absolutely delighted. It gets better and better. It's very strange, and this isn't a trite sort of remark, it really is bloody marvellous.

*How does it get better and better?*

Ah ... about five or six strands to this. I think that companionship is a marvellous thing. And that's a little bit self-seeking, because one is looking ahead and thinking, 'Gee, wouldn't it be frightful to go on and on if you had no companionship?' And if you have love as well, that's even better; that's terrific. But I think that companionship and health come first on the list. Then there's more time; more time for everything. Linked up with that is the fact that it's marvellous not to feel you've got to get to an office by a given time. I was an office chap. It's even more marvellous to realise that you haven't got to be polite to lots of people. I don't mean you want to be rude; but when you're retired, there aren't lots of people to whom you *have* to be polite all the time. It's also idly satisfying to realise you don't have to persuade a lot of people to agree with what you want to do. You're your own man or woman. So, companionship, health, time, taking your own decisions—they're part of the answer.

Something else I specially like is that if one is very lucky—and we've been lucky—you get to know a lot of young people. And if you are even luckier they somehow like you. The point of this being that, when you are with them, you realise that they look forward. They don't look back. Sometimes, they don't even look at the present. A lot of people of my age are looking back, plus they have a heavy involvement with the immediate present—'Have you got the sausages for tea?'

*And you don't do that?*

No, although in the case of food I look forward madly to every single meal. I adore food now much more than I've ever done in my life. I like all the things about being part of preparing it. This is all tied up with having time and having companionship. I'd hate to prepare a marvellous meal all on my own for myself; that would be terrible.

*Were you conscious of virility, looks, and so on when you were a young man?*

I always thought—and still think—that I'm absolutely a non-starter there. I used to think it was marvellous to meet and see beautiful people, whether they were male or female.

*How have you felt about changes in your physical appearance?*

I was in the greengrocer's the other day, and I happened to look at a display of fruit and noticed that it had an angled-mirror backing. I looked at it, and found that I had a bald spot on the top of my head. It's ridiculous. What does it matter? But I was absolutely horrified! Occasionally, I feel as if I need ironing from top to bottom—all those wrinkles and creases and folds.

*Do you feel your wrinkles are ugly, or do you feel quite affectionate about them?*

I just try to disregard them. And if somebody doesn't like them, well, too bad. I'm much more likely to be conscious of other people's bodies. My own happens to be a dead loss; but, never mind. I've always brushed my hair, and that sort of thing, and I try and look neat and tidy.

*Are you equally tolerant and accepting about the changes in your partner?*

Absolutely, but I'm absolutely delighted that she manages to look a good ten or fifteen years younger than she actually is. I think she's much better looking, and her skin is much better and all that sort of thing, than lots of the people we know who are her age. I'm aware that she is older now. Of course I am. But it hasn't really got much to do with it, because if you have this companionship and love, it's just so nice to be together. There was a great moment the other day when I was in my room writing, and my wife suddenly came in. She was wearing a woolly sweater and a pair of these marvellously jazzy, highly coloured, dizzy-looking leggings; so quite suddenly there were the whole of her long legs, which I don't normally look at. She's usually dressed in such a way that you like the whole of her outfit. Or you're swimming, and you've got no clothes on, and you like the whole of that. I'd never before directed my attention solely to these marvellous legs. I thought it was very funny.

*What has happened to your attitudes towards sex and your own sexuality?*

I've always been attracted to women, and obviously particularly to young women because they're usually so nice to look at, and they're fun and they're jolly. But as you get older you appreciate all that more and more; it's marvellous. If there is any advice you can give to anybody who's worried about becoming fifty: don't think that sex stops, and don't let it stop. When you get to approaching sixty, exactly the same. When you're approaching seventy, exactly the same. And I suspect the same advice when you are approaching eighty!

Now, maybe there are lots of people who aren't orientated this way. I don't mean that I'm a sort of sex maniac—five times a week and six times on Saturday. No, but sex is definitely a part of life, and it goes on getting better. It's never monotonous, and I think that's marvellous. I don't know what other men think. One gets the impression that in their raging fifties some men get sex-mad, but unaccompanied by feelings—the late-middle-age thing. I think that perhaps I'm lucky, I don't know, but I very much appreciate all sorts and kinds of women, young women, girls. Certainly, to me they're 'sexy,' but I don't think of myself being sexy with them. For instance, take a simple example: we've got a heated outdoor spa pool, and most people strip off when they go into that, and it's all good fun. It's also very nice to look at, but it's nothing to do with sex!

*Dick, are there any disadvantages in getting older?*

Yes, there are some, but in nearly every case they have an opposite plus. Here's a silly example. One's memory goes a bit. Take, for instance, books—and I happen to mirror in this exactly what my friend Nigel Nicolson feels and has written—but it's also me. It's marvellous to say, 'Ah, I remember that book; I'd love to read that again.' But you can't remember the characters; you certainly can't remember the denouement; and so it's wonderful that you get a second go of discovery and pleasure. It's a disadvantage, in that it's a bore for other people if your memory is bad, and I'm sure mine slips a bit. I find that what I tend to rationalise as 'tunnel vision' is also a bit of a bore. If I go into a room to look for something, I'll look for that; but if somebody shouts out to look for something else, I don't see it. And yet it's there when I go back into the room. How could I have missed it? This is irritating to other people. Another annoying thing, although it doesn't worry me so much, is getting a bit deaf. There's a flip-side to that. You can mis-hear the most marvellous things, unbelievably funny things you can *think* you've heard.

Aches and pains? Yes, at the moment, tremendous aches and pains, because I had a replacement hip for nine years and then had to have another one. So that's a bore, but there again there are many people much wiser than I who've said for centuries, 'When it stops, it's marvellous.' For instance, I can still sit down without pain. I can still lie down without pain. Wonderful. Bloody awful in between, sometimes. But super when it stops. I'm not trying to be clever. It's a real fact: sink into a chair and think, 'Gee, isn't that marvellous!'

*Do you ever get frightened about getting older?*

I'm apprehensive about becoming more of a bore. For instance, at my age, you can't see somebody you haven't seen for five or six months and start telling a story without having to check if you've told it before. But the whole point about telling stories is merely to get other people to talk to you. They're kick-starters. I don't think they should be show-off things. If you make people laugh, they'll tell you something back.

*Do you think you're more tolerant?*

Yes, I am sure I am more tolerant. But there are things of which I am intolerant.

*Such as?*

Spelling, grammar, no apostrophe in 'French's Forest': that sort of thing. ABC newsreaders who get names wrong: not tricky names; ordinary names. I'm intolerant of that because I feel it's unprofessional. I'm not tolerant of bad manners, although you have to put up with them. And the moment the bad-mannered people are gone, boy does one tear them to shreds!

*How about wisdom?*

A lot of the young friends we've got give the impression of thinking that what one has to say is wise. But I think it's experience, rather than actual wisdom. I'm not quite sure what wisdom is—it's something inherent, right inside, but experience is something that's been put inside you by what you've gone through.

*Dick, we talked about fear of getting older. What about fear of death?*

Um, I don't want to die because I am enjoying life so much. I really love it. I think it's marvellous. On the other hand, clearly one's going to die; so there's no point in fussing. What, I think, confuses the whole thing is the difference in the passage of time: the passage of time in a day, and the passage of time in a week. A day can go endlessly slowly;

but come Friday night, where the hell did that week go? It's gone. So if we are talking about death, I'm very keen that the weeks should somehow pass a little more slowly, but the days sometimes should pass a bit more quickly. I don't want to do the dying bit, not at all. A sudden heart attack, plane crash if we could both be together—that would be okay. But I don't want to do all that awful, long, drawn-out torture, pain, agony stuff. Except, I think you could put up with it if you didn't want to die because of wanting to get the most you could out of what was left.

*Do you think that you should be allowed to take your own life if you wish?*
Yes, absolutely, under all kinds of conditions of the sensible Dutch kind. I think it's intolerable that other people should demand that you suffer. It's got no part of my life at all, no part of my thinking.

*You have talked about your love and companionship with your wife. Are you frightened that she might die before you?*
Absolutely. Major fear. Absolutely major. Tempered by two things. One, that I'd hate it for *her* if I died first, because I think that although she is wonderfully self-contained and marvellously strong, I think it would be bloody awful for anybody to lose the day-to-day contact—however irritating—that you've become so used to. The other tempering factor is that—and I wouldn't want to impose on her at all—I now have my younger daughter who has emigrated, and lives here in Sydney. That would be a great comfort, but one would have to be very, very careful not to be a bore, and not to impose or demand. Fortunately, we are very fond of each other; so that would be a help but, oh, I would hate it. That's why we both agree that the joint plane crash is the ideal if selfish solution.

*Do you think there is any life after death?*
I simply don't. I think you're here for a good run. You're physical. You crumble, you die, and that's it. Now, having said that, there is a wavy sort of difficulty, partly because it seems extraordinary that with people who've done wonderful things, and who've influenced people quite marvellously, that their influence shouldn't go on.

*So does this worry you?*

It infuriates me. If you're lucky enough to have fun, if you're lucky enough to have an interesting time, if you're lucky enough to be the sort of person who's got masses more to achieve, life is all too short. Quite ludicrously, desperately short. Of course, I understand that's the sort of argument for my being wrong, and maybe there is something afterwards. But I can't see it. All that stuff about coming back as a seagull, I think that's absurd.

*How would you like to be remembered?*

Ah ... I've never thought about that ... um ... perhaps as somebody who was interested enough in other people, and particularly younger people, to try to be helpful to them. There's no great achievement I've got to be remembered for, none of that, and so my answer is a bit waffly; but I think that's what I feel. Of course, it's much easier to do when you're retired, and getting older, because you have time. One realises, of course, that it's a permanently renewing cycle. You know them when they haven't got anybody, and then you meet the person they've got, and then you know them when they're married, and then they have a baby, and then one's less needed. But by that time you've inevitably met some other 'youngies', and so the cycle goes on and on. I think it's good fun. And what's very fortunate is that, although my wife is far better educated than I am, she has always spent her professional life with young people; because she was a fashion editor for many years, and that meant constantly dealing with young people. And so she likes being good at helping them. She gets a bit narked if there are too many, and they interrupt her own writing, but that's understandable.

*How do you feel about what's happening in the world now? Do you think we are any better as human beings than we were two or more thousand years ago?*

I've got three things about this. One is that I am absolutely sickened by violence. I am sickened by war. I can't bear to think that all these terrible things go on, being done by people to other people. It really upsets me very badly, and there's nothing I can do about it. Secondly, I think it's quite splendid that there are so many people who do *wonderful* things. I find that most inspiring. And thirdly, I am heavily in favour of women having the greater responsibility in more fields, and the greater power. I've said responsibility first, power second, and that's because men have made a real muck of so many things. It's encouraging that there are these new emerging women in important positions. One just hopes they really have the influence, and are allowed to go on having it.

*Have you any advice to people who are getting older?*
Mental activities really are important. They can be anything: work, theatre, crosswords, writing, reading, but *do* it. Physical activities are not top of my list of important points, but you've got to do *something*. It's worth walking, it's worth maintaining your garden, it's worth swimming, it's worth exercising—if only to keep your health. And perhaps some funny suggestions: I think it's very important to keep on going out. That need not mean whacking great holidays costing hundreds or thousands of dollars. It may mean deliberately going into Sydney one day a week, or going for a walk two days a week. You must not let yourself become sealed up in your home, no matter how grand it may be (not that ours is).

Saying what one thinks, that's a great thing about getting older: you don't have to look over your shoulder. And there is writing real letters; it's marvellous to have time for them, and to have somebody who's prepared to accept them, ten pages, full of thoughts, impressions and ideas, not just what you did yesterday. Try to do new things sometimes; don't get in a rut. A last small point: it's very nice feeling better after you've had an afternoon nap; it may be short, but you wake up feeling wonderful.

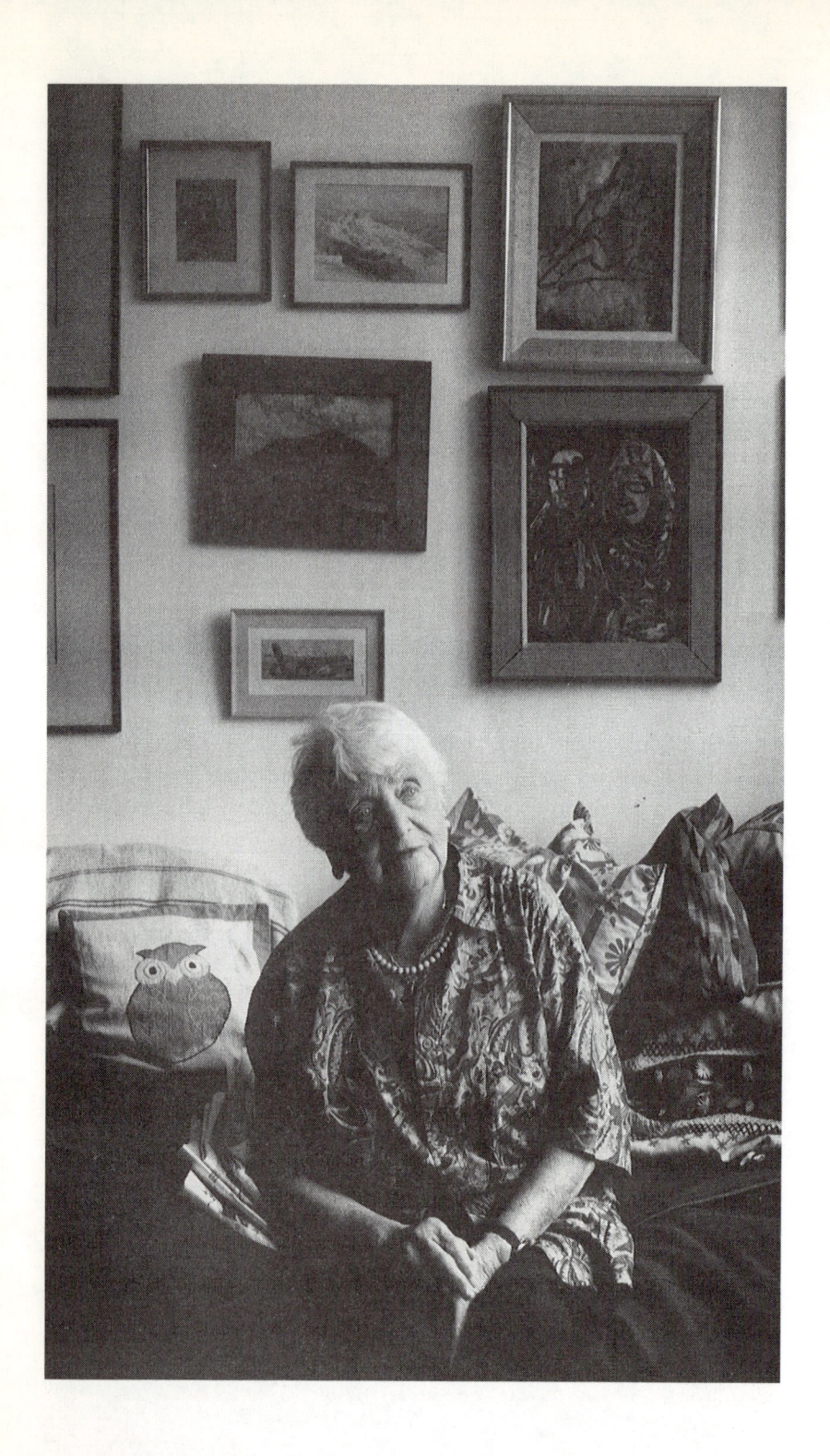

# Barbara Wace
*I find the world terribly interesting*

Barbara Wace was the first British woman to report on the Allied invasion of Europe in the last world war. In Brest, when somebody took her clothes, her despatch, 'Lost skirt, Brest fallen', caused much merriment in the offices of Associated Press. Now in her mid-eighties, Wace is still working as a journalist and still travelling. In the last two years, she has been in China, Hongkong, Hungary, Romania, Russia, Italy, Norway, the United States, Canada, Outer Mongolia, and Ghana. She is also writing her memoirs.

Barbara Wace was born in Kent into an Army family on 4 August 1907. She spent much of her childhood in Germany while her father was head of the Boundary Commission of the Saar, which decided on the Franco-German border after the First World War. She first trained as a typist, and took a job with the British Embassy in Berlin, where she was working at the time of the 1936 Olympics. In 1940, she set up the British Information Service in Washington, and then moved to New York and San Francisco to establish similar bureaux. She joined American Associated Press after she returned to London in 1942. Ever since then she has lived in or near Fleet Street, and is a Freeman of the City of London.

Her small flat constantly overflows with people of vastly diverse backgrounds and ages, most of whom she feeds and looks after. On her eighty-fourth birthday she had over seventy people to a party which lasted until three in the morning; the oldest guest was ninety-four, and the youngest was two. On her eighty-fifth, she escaped to Italy; she said she wanted not to think about it.

I look at myself in the mirror as seldom as I can, and I hate photographs of myself. I never like to accept that's what I really look like. I have a couple of pictures on my pinboard looking absolutely lovely in a bathing suit. I look at those sometimes, and it makes me feel much better.

*Do you ever feel like your mother?*

No. I wish I did. I think my mother was much more sensible. My mother's generation weren't so puzzled. She lived a long time; both of them did, Daddy lived until he was about eighty-seven. Mother accepted her age more, and she expected that people would help her, and be nice and kind when she was old. I don't expect it, because people aren't very.

*Do you let people help you?*

[Laughs] I find that people try and do all sorts of things you don't want, like carry your bag when it's quite light. But there are very few people you can really rely on who are going to ring up to see if you're not dead in your bed—and haven't been dead for three weeks. I'm sounding bitter, and I'm not bitter, but we all used to ring aunt Agnes once a week to make sure she was all right. Nobody rings me up, and I could be dead in my bed. I'm not lonely. Lots of people are fond of me, but they don't think it's necessary to check on me.

*So is there a price to pay for independence?*

Yes, definitely. I'd rather be independent, because I don't like being fussed around. I'd like to go on as long as I can the way I always have, listening to the news and being a part of everything.

*Do you find that people's expectations of old age put restrictions on you?*

No. Daphne, my sister, who's seventy-seven, exploded to me on the phone the other day when I'd said something to her about trying to come down for lunch: she said most people of our age aren't expected to do nearly as much.

*How do you cope with physical restraints?*

Not being able to move around with this silly gammy knee I have, and not being able to run, irritates me. I miscalculate. I think I'm going to get everywhere faster than I do, because I go slower. I find it very irritating to be wobbly, and I take a stick. Before I went to Mongolia, this friend said, 'Take a stick.' And I said, 'I can't possibly. I've got a suitcase in one hand and my cameras in the other; there's no room for a stick.' She said, 'You *must* take a stick.' And because she was so dominating about it, I took a stick. And it was the best advice—because if you signal to people, they know you need help. But I don't want to be fussed over too much. It's nice if you find someone who understands that what you want is a shoulder; you don't want a wobbly hand. People are awfully silly. They aren't very helpful. They try to be, but half the time they're a damned nuisance.

*Do you feel mentally slower?*
I don't think I'm mentally slower, because I've never had a particularly disciplined life. But I do find it very depressing that there's such a lot of things that I just don't understand at all and I don't think it's worth my trying. For instance, all that stuff with computers. It's cut me off from a lot of very young people, because I can't play computer games and they get furious with me.

I was brought up to think I wasn't any good at anything do to with science and with money. That was partly from mother, because my father was very good at that. He was an engineer. I always remember my mother crying at the accounts; she cried every week, because she got into a muddle. So I always felt I didn't want to learn.

*Are you conscious a lot of the time of being old?*
Yes, because I ache. Let me think about that a bit more. Yes, because some people treat you as if you are old. The people who don't treat you as if you are old are the really young people. It's the people who are your age that are the worst.

*Sorry about that! Do you find you are less concerned to be polite than you were when you were younger?*
I knew you'd ask me questions I haven't had time to think about. I think that I no longer want to be liked as much by everybody, therefore I don't mind as much saying something that's going to upset somebody. It's a failing of mine that I wanted everybody to like me. That I'd be upset if the bus conductor wasn't nice when I got on the bus, and I'd spend a long time jollying him along so when I got off I'd think, 'Well,

he liked me in the end.' I don't do that as much as I used to.

*How do you like to be treated?*

People have got to accept that you're old, and treat you sensibly. Just because you're lively in conversation doesn't mean you can run up the stairs, and it's useful that people don't try and push you when you're going down the stairs. But there's no reason why you shouldn't be mentally exactly like everybody who's young.

*But if people see you with a stick and notice your physical limitations, do they also think you have mental limitations?*

Not people who know me; but sometimes others, when they see the stick, they're absolutely astounded that you aren't an old woman with no new ideas. I think that young people are astounded that you are still interested in what they're interested in, and it pleases them.

*I find that interesting, because it gets back to the fact that we do have expectations of what people are supposed to be like.*

I get irritated with even the young, because if I talk about dying—if they are having supper with me—and I say, 'Is that the picture you would like me to leave you?' they all say, 'Oh, don't talk about it.' But why not talk about it? It's a very interesting thing that's going to happen to you; perhaps the only interesting thing after you're a certain age. I'm not being morbid. I'm planning out the next year, which may very well include that I may die. And, anyway, I want to get tidied up.

*I've noticed that when you say you're 'shutting the door' on certain countries, people also get irritated.*

Yes, that's right. You can't go on seeing the whole world if you've only got a certain amount of time. For instance, I've decided not to go to South America, because I haven't time to see South America. I'd rather go back to a few places and tidy them up. But I don't think that's morbid. I think that's sensible.

*Are you scared of dying?*

I'm not scared of death itself. I think it's frightfully interesting, don't you? I want to know what happens. I think everybody is scared of *how* they die. I don't see how you could not be, in case it's painful and an illness, and in case you can't look after yourself and you're going to be an awful bore. However much people love you, if you take ages dying it's terrible for the family.

*Do you get angry because, for a great many people, the end of their lives can be both painful and ignominious?*
I don't feel angry. I just feel apprehensive. I don't know who to be angry with! I suppose if you really believed in God, you'd be angry with God. But I'm not sure that I really believe in God.

*Would it be easier if you did believe in God?*
No. I'm quite happy to be with an open mind. I think people who do believe totally in God are happier, but I don't see that there's any proof. I'm certainly not an atheist. Anything could be true. I like to go to church: I love the music, I like the old hymns, I like the words of the Bible, I like the feeling that everybody welcomes you when you go there. I go to evening service, but I couldn't go to communion, and I can't say the creed. I don't believe it, but I don't disbelieve it. I don't think any of the things in the Bible are any more wonderful than any of the scientific things I don't understand. It seems to me there could be some sort of God, or there could be an after-life. I haven't really thought it through. But I still find the fact of going to church comforting, and I suppose that's because I went to church with my family. Mother didn't really believe it, either. My father believed it all explicitly. He read every bit of the Bible.

*Are there things you regret in your life?*
No. I don't regret much in my life. But if I had my life over again I wouldn't do it just the same. Everybody says they would, but I wouldn't. I was very swallowed up by my family problems for a while, and I think I wouldn't be as nice to some people as I was. But that's not a very kind attitude!

*How much of that was because you weren't married?*
Oh, yes. Because if you are married you've got such a good excuse—you've got a husband, a family—but the single woman then was seen as being available to help everyone.

*What changes have you seen occur for single women?*
I think people would believe you more now if you said you'd chosen

to be single, whereas when I was young nobody would believe you,. And anyway, maybe most people do want to be married and have a family.

*Did you?*

Of course I did; of course I did.

*But you made a decision not to?*

No, I didn't make a decision. It was made for me. I tried to make someone marry me, and he didn't. The only thing is that he didn't marry anybody else, so that was good!

*But you could have married other people?*

Oh yes, but I didn't want second best. Would you? I think you go for what you want, and if you don't get it you're not a martyr. But what's better now is that people get married when they're much older. In my day, you were on the shelf if you were twenty-five and not married. I remember thinking my sister would be on the shelf and no chance of getting married if she didn't hurry up. And that's totally changed. Also, you don't feel ludicrous any more these days, behaving young when you're old. I remember when somebody made a pass at me on a ship in Yugoslavia just after the war, turning on him and saying, 'Don't make a pass at me, I'm over forty, it's ridiculous.' And he didn't. He went away horrified to think I was forty.

But that doesn't exist any more, does it? People have affairs when they're fifty and sixty, and nobody laughs at them. It's totally changed. Whereas my grandmother's mother put on a mob cap at thirty, and never got up again. She had a bachelor son who used to get her up for lunch, lift her out of bed and take her on the verandah, and that's all she did. People walked right into old age. There's still a side of me that thinks there is something ludicrous about anyone over the age of sixty being in love. Yet I've seen people in love; and I think I could be, too.

*I remember a friend of mine who is nearly fifty, saying rather sadly that nobody's going to fall head over heels in love with her any more, the way they might have when she was younger. Men aren't going to follow her down the street.*

Yes, and if you do have something physical that is still good, people say, 'My, you have the bluest eyes I've ever seen'—as if it's the only thing I've got left.

*Lots of people's blue eyes fade. Yours haven't.*
No, mine haven't. They haven't moved people very much, though!

*What other major changes for women have occurred in your life-time?*
I think the big one is that you can have an interesting life and not be married. I wanted to go to university. My mother said, 'If you go to university, you'll be a highbrow, and the men won't like you.' And everything you wanted in life when you were quite young circled around the idea that you would be married, and that some man would like you. That isn't the case nowadays. All these young women have careers of their own.

*In spite of the attitudes to women which you grew up with, you succeeded as a journalist who's worked around the world in some very interesting political situations.*
Well, my father's job was the first appointment with the League of Nations as president of the Bounty Commission of the Saar. We had our own mess, and it had six nationalities in it. So I wasn't bought up with a steady English background at all. I had my thirteenth birthday in Saar Brucken, and I have a picture of me sitting on the knee of a Japanese. We were brought up thinking it was one world.

*You were also brought up to think there were certain things that women couldn't do, but you broke through that.*
Up to a point. I think that sometimes women try to do things that they don't do terribly well. That's probably the wrong attitude. but I still have it a bit. I always remember you saying, 'If men can do it, I can do it.' I don't feel like that. I think there are things that men do much better; let 'em do it, like boring things—knowing about electricity. I don't want to. I'm still very old-fashioned that way and lazy, I suppose.

*Have you ever been held back in your work because you were a woman?*
No, but I could have been in the AAP (American Associated Press). The men were very jealous when I went to Normandy during the war; but they hadn't any reason to be, because it had to be a woman that went over to the WACS. I remember one man saying, 'You did awfully

well; you covered it just like a man.' I was awfully careful never to stress that I was a woman. I signed, 'B Wace' on the whole, and I very seldom did a story that was written from the point of view of a woman; which was different; because most of the women war correspondents stressed the fact that they were a woman, and I was very careful not to, which was probably very stupid—because I wanted the men to like me.

*Would you rather not have had that attitude?*
I think it's a weakness.

*While you were working as a war correspondent, were you frightened?*
Yes, most of the things I've done in life to do with work, I've mostly let the tail of the dog wag me. I didn't plan to be a journalist. I didn't in the least want to be. I came home from America where I'd escaped the blitz, and I thought, 'Now I've got to go and work in a factory.' So I volunteered, and the Ministry of Labour said, 'Oh no, get yourself a job with the Americans.' And that was a very sensible thing, because there weren't any English people that knew Americans. It was the beginning of the war, and there hadn't been many over. I went to Normandy quite by mistake, because they brought a girl over specially for the invasion, and she didn't answer the phone the night they rang up. You couldn't be warned ahead; so they got me about midnight, and I was gone by three in the morning.

*You lived in Germany before the war and saw the rise of fascism with its appalling consequences. Do you think the world is now a better place?*
It can't be, because the same things are starting to happen again. I do feel that a lot of things are better, but a lot of things are worse. And even in countries where it seems safe, isn't there more commercial cheating? Isn't there more government secrecy? Or am I wrong? I feel there's a lot of evil around in London. I feel the yuppies don't care about anything; I don't like the yuppies very much.

*Do you think you are wiser now that you are older?*
I feel that I'm wiser, but I'm not sure that what I say is wiser. I think I interfere less with people, especially young people. I let them talk, and I don't try and influence them as much as I used to. But whether that's wiser or whether that's lazy, I don't know.

*Why do you think that is?*

Because you learn from experience that you can't really change people; that they are going to do what they want, and it's better to stay close to them and go along with what they're doing than confront them. You will lose them if you confront them.

*You've always had lots of young people around you. Has this been by choice?*

Yes, definitely. I'm nice to them because I want everyone to like me. I don't want to be disliked.

*Yes, except that's presenting a picture of a dear sweet old lady rushing around with tea and sympathy, and you're not like that. You can be quite tart, yet young people love coming to you.*

I think I've always felt that older people should be closer to young people. Once I faced the fact that I probably wasn't going to have children, then I think I was happy to have a share of other people's children. I've enjoyed other people's children very much; and when they grow up, then I know their children; and now their children's children.

*And children really do want to come—I am thinking of my children.*

I think children do need an outside friend. I suppose it sounds a sloppy thing to say, but every family needs outside grown-ups. There's always a period when your mother knows too much about you; so if you can talk to somebody else who knows a bit about you, but not too much, it's a relief. I'm very grateful to the young people I know. They keep me alive.

*What about people from your own childhood?*

Yes. I remember my grandmother who was very dominating, granny Sim. She was interested in everything. She was a selfish old lady and bossy, but she opened a lot of sides of life to me. She taught me about music and about other things. I don't remember old people being terribly wise—they were always supposed to be. They often seemed to be wrong to me.

*Your mother was a very loving and open person. Do you think she influenced you?*

Yes, definitely. My mother influenced my sister and me. Everything that I think of as a rule of life—and I mostly say them to myself—were things that mother said, and they were very simple. She must have been influenced by some old nanny, because I find myself ruling my life by nursery rhymes: like, 'Do the thing that's nearest, though its hard at times, Helping when you meet them, lame dogs over stiles', or something like that!

*What do you remember about your mother?*
Her little weaknesses more than anything else. I remember her as immensely sympathetic and immensely loving, but really rather muddly. I always remember we used to get so cross with her because she used to have egg on her dressing-gown when she had breakfast in bed; and now I find I've got egg on my dressing-gown. I regret being tough with her sometimes, and I remember her with great affection.

*I also remember going to see her when she was ninety-one, and it was Carnaby Road time, Flower Power, Mods and Winklepickers, and she was talking about it all with enormous enthusiasm and delight.*
Yes, mother was tremendously interested in everything right up until she died, and I think that's very important. I remember when she was literally dying, showing her a picture of Chichester; and she couldn't speak, but she saw the picture and she pointed and tried to say something about it. So that right up to the last minute she was interested in what was going on. I think that has influenced me very much. She was always terribly interested in people; she always wanted to meet new people. It fascinates me that a lot of people don't want to see new people. I want to see new people all the time. I want to keep my old friends, but I want to meet new ones, too.

*Do you plan your life now that you're older?*
No, because I always think that something interesting might turn up now. Except I am sitting here in Italy, and I've decided that I will change. I will be wiser, and not get so tired, and not have so many people in, and not spend so much money. I would like to do that, but I won't. You know I won't [laughs]. I see myself sitting there quietly at my desk, but ... I think you can't do so much work when you get old, I do feel that. I'm not morbid; I'm not going to die, but I do feel

that I'm not going to be as good next year as I am this. So if I want to go somewhere next year, I'd better hurry up and go, because the year after that I may be in a wheel chair or my brain may go.

*Does that worry you?*
Yes. There are quite a lot of things I still want to do.

*I wonder if we do change, or if we just kid ourselves?*
I think you remain essentially the same, except I do realise now that I get awfully tired. And if you get awfully tired you don't cook the meal very well, you're rather cross to everybody, you might get ill. And therefore I am trying to be a bit more sensible about how I spend my energies. So, I'm saying your energies do go a bit, but I think you stay essentially the same. My feeling is that the longer you can stay the same, the better you are—because what's the good of stopping things if you don't have to, and you like what you're doing?

*So is it a matter of accepting yourself as you now are?*
I think one of the things that is difficult when you get old is the feeling that you're no longer any use to anybody. But I think if you don't get too tired you still are of use, because you're still a nice place for people to come. I am still some use to young people.

*Was that a strong message from your mother or your father, that you had a responsibility in life to be useful?*
Yes. I think mother, and father up to a point. They thought that you aren't here for nothing. It must be awful to be of no use, and nobody to need you. Everybody needs to be needed.

*The fact that you are confronting a limited span of time, how does that affect you?*
I feel, 'Oh God, there's not much time left.' I find the world terribly interesting. I don't want to go away.